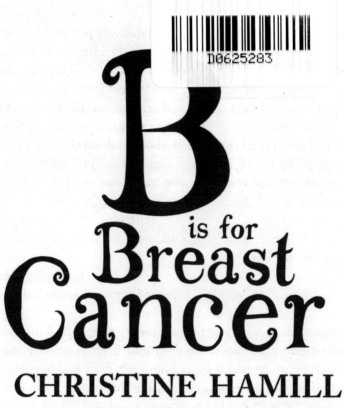

B is for Breast Cancer

CHRISTINE HAMILL

From anxiety to recovery and everything
in between – a beginner's guide

piatkus

PIATKUS

First published in Great Britain in 2014 by Piatkus

A CIP catalogue record for this book
is available from the British Library.

ISBN 978-0-349-40134-8

Typeset in Minion by M Rules
Printed and bound in Great Britain by
Clays Ltd St Ives plc

Papers used by Piatkus are from well-managed forests
and other responsible sources.

MIX
Paper from
responsible sources
FSC
www.fsc.org   FSC® C104740

Piatkus
An imprint of
Little, Brown Book Group
100 Victoria Embankment
London EC4Y 0DY

An Hachette UK Company
www.hachette.co.uk

www.piatkus.co.uk

In memory of Olive

About the Author

Christine Hamill studied English literature at university in the 1980s before working in the arts as a gallery manager and an administrator on an arts magazine. She then became a teacher, working in Spain and England, before teaching full time at a college in Northern Ireland. Christine was diagnosed with breast cancer and wrote this book while having treatment. She has also written a novel for children. Christine lives in Belfast with her son.

If you were not a worrier before being
diagnosed with cancer, you will be afterwards.
Stay sane. Read this. It helps to know you are not alone.

This is not a medical guide.

Contents

Contents

Acknowledgements

Thanks to everyone who helped make this book possible: to Eilish, for taking the time to read it and comment; to my agent Eve White, who read the manuscript and 'got it' straight away; to everyone at Little, Brown, especially Anne Lawrance and Jillian Stewart, for their enthusiasm and expertise; and to my copyeditor, the very patient Anne Newman.

Thanks also go to Cancer Focus Northern Ireland for supporting me (although I prefer not to single anyone out, I would like to remember counsellor Dorothy Smallwoods, now sadly passed away); to Tony Cook of abctales.com, who loved this book from the start and never stopped encouraging me; to Callan for countless cups of tea; and to Janey, just for being Janey.

I would also like to remember my parents who are mentioned in this book but who passed away before it was published.

Introduction

Whose boob is it anyway?

Having breast cancer is a bit like being pregnant except, of course, you're miserable and don't have a cute baby to look forward to at the end of it. Think of the similarities: the breast pain, the sleepless nights, the anxiety, the constant bursting into tears, the overwhelming immobilising fatigue, the forgetfulness, the endless examinations, the hormonal maelstrom. See what I mean?

Of course, whereas pregnancy lasts only nine glorious, slow-moving months, cancer will never leave you, even when you have been cured. That sounds like a life sentence of misery, but oddly, it isn't. There are things to laugh about with cancer, even in the face of grief. That is why I started writing this A to Z, as an antidote to all the sadness and mystery that surround cancer.

The first thing that struck me about cancer, right from day

one, was that I seemed to become public property. Anyone who has ever been pregnant will remember that feeling of being taken over: suddenly everyone, including complete strangers, knows better than you how to care for your unborn baby. They will walk up to you and touch your bump, then tell you what to eat, what to drink, how much exercise to take, berating you when you go wrong. And, of course, they will tell you their own horror stories. Cancer is no different: as soon as you reveal your diagnosis, your relationship with the world changes. People feel empowered to discuss your body and your life without your say-so, and you will find people you don't know very well (and never much liked) discussing your malignant breasts as if they were teacups. I am convinced that this same level of audience participation would not be acceptable if it were a man's testicles in question. I have tried to substantiate this hypothesis, but no one seemed prepared to talk about it – which kind of proves my point. (Likewise, I cannot imagine a situation where men were referred to the Testicle Care Unit.)

When I was diagnosed with cancer I felt this sense of being taken over acutely and it made me feel like I no longer had much control over my life. This is a feeling that can be compounded by the knowledge that your doctors know more about your condition than you do, and you can't help sitting there wondering, What are they not telling me? And don't be surprised if you come over all proprietorial: even though I desperately wanted to be rid of the cancer, I did find myself thinking more than once, Whose boobs are these, anyway? This is my body, my boob, my lump; surely I should be the one who is in possession of all the facts. I know that some women won't want to know about their cancer or their treatment (and I suppose they should have this right), but I did. Also, apparently, around eight in ten breast cancers are diagnosed in women aged fifty and over. This means that they have been in control of their lives and bodies for some considerable period of time. I can't be the only person who isn't ready to abdicate control. And I can't be the only one who knew diddly squat about cancer. Never before have I felt like such a dunce. I was completely clueless. I had so many questions my brain ached: Why? How? What? And again, Why? But sometimes it felt like the answers were just cosy clichés and chirpy sound bites about positive mental attitude. So your best bet, it seems, is to go easy on the questions and to stay silently, stubbornly positive. And that's fine, if you can. If you can't, read on . . .

A is for anxiety

Cancer and anxiety go together like New Year's Eve and Auld Lang Syne, but without the drunken snogging. They are best friends, so you better get used to it.

Take note: anxiety can make you do strange things, like asking your babysitter to feel your boob. Yes, I actually did that. There I was, chatting away to my babysitter when I put my hand up to my armpit and found a pea-sized lump and immediately asked her to have a feel. It occurs to me that you could be arrested for less, so I should tell you that my babysitter is an adult and she is also a friend. Anyway, she said no (actually, she screeched it) and scurried from the house, leaving me to my anxiety. Anxiety about taking time off work to get it checked out; anxiety about feeling foolish and wasting everyone's time; anxiety about not being able to locate the lump for the doctor; anxiety about taking my kit off and having my breast kneaded by a complete stranger, or worse, someone I already knew in a fully clothed capacity, like the GP I only see when my son has a cough; anxiety about which shade of wood to choose for my coffin. The list goes on.

Even when you are almost convinced, as I was, that they will detect nothing more than a time-wasting little cyst, there will still be an undercurrent of anxiety: the *what-if* factor. But this is good. Anxiety is good; don't let anyone tell you otherwise. It proves beyond doubt that you are sane and sensible and prepared to defend yourself. Doctors don't like anxiety; doctors like anxiolytics (tranquillisers to you and me). These are drugs that take your anxiety away and make you feel perfectly calm in the face of chaos. Think back to your school days and to Rudyard Kipling's 'If':

> If you can keep your head when all about you
> Are losing theirs and blaming it on you . . .
> Yours is the Earth and everything that's in it,

Now think of the wag who rewrote it thus:

> If you can keep your head while all about you
> Are losing theirs – you have assessed the situation
>   incorrectly.

I'm with the wag. You'd be mad not to feel anxious at a time like this. Of course, it would be detrimental to your health and relationships to be in a state of high alert all of the time, and so for some people, some of the time, medication may be a good thing, especially if your anxiety is interfering with your actual functioning. I, however, found that I could function quite well and be anxious at the same time. I can worry, cry, bite my nails, wring my hands and gnash my teeth while preparing dinner, doing the ironing or making a packed lunch for my son. I experienced high anxiety at the point of diagnosis, but this dissipated over time, returning only in sporadic outbursts, like guerrilla warfare, until eventually it burned down to a low-grade irritant. Get used to your anxiety; it is not going away. So don't think of it as the enemy; think of it more as your personal early-warning system, urging you to get that twinge in your neck seen by the doctor, making sure you check your body for odd changes, wagging a finger at you when you stray from your born-again healthy-eating regime. Anxiety shows you care about yourself. Embrace it.

During this time your anxiety may lead you to contemplate a worst-case scenario. Don't panic. Somehow, just contemplating the worst means that your prognosis and treatment plan might come as less of a shock than if you'd gone nonchalantly about thinking, Nothing can happen to me, I am indestructible; because we are none of us indestructible.

I allowed myself a glimpse of the worst right at the start and then I shut it away. They will tell you that a positive mindset is crucial to recovery (see page 138), and I am sure it is, but realism is important too. My sister died after surgery to a tumour on her brain when she was three years younger than I am now. My maternal aunt died of breast cancer and her daughter began chemotherapy to reduce a breast tumour one month before my diagnosis, so I never felt I could afford myself the luxury of thinking it couldn't happen to me. If you do take a peek at the unthinkable, make it brief, use the fear to fix up your will and sort out your affairs (see page 14), then shut your eyes to it and get on with the business of being positive.

If you are not feeling anxiety, go straight to D for denial.

A is for axilla

Axilla is what medical folk call your armpit. *The Collins Concise Dictionary* says it's the technical term for the armpit, comes from Latin and was first used in English in the seventeenth century. Who'd have guessed? And there I was thinking the correct term was oxter. In all my forty-five semi-literate years I never once came across the term axilla; not once in all those *ER*-watching hours did I ever hear George Clooney say, 'Mighty fine axilla you have there, mam!' Who ever heard of anyone going off to shave their axillas – or should that be axillum? (No, it's axillae – I just checked.) So taken aback was I by my lack of knowledge that I couldn't even bear to ask anyone what it meant. I needn't have worried though, as I received reams of literature telling me all about the axilla and breast cancer.

The lump I found was in the axilla tail. I tried very hard to concentrate as the doctor was telling me this, but I was so distracted by the idea of having a tail in this part of my anatomy that I couldn't focus. I started imagining my armpit as a small predatory animal eating me alive. A kind of savage, furry dormouse. I began to fear my armpit almost as much as I feared the suspect breast. Then I perked up; if the lump was in my armpit it couldn't be breast cancer, could it? Armpit cancer doesn't have the same ring to it. I liked it – who ever heard of anyone dying of armpit cancer? Anyway, when I refocused on what the doctor was saying I realised she was talking about the tail end of the breast tissue that extends down into the armpit, and that if anything was eating me alive it was definitely my breast. As it turned out, I needn't have exerted myself with this line of thought because on examination they found a second lump lurking just behind the nipple. Oxter, axilla, armpit, schmarmpit, it didn't matter any more.

Incidentally, I just checked oxter in the dictionary and it is Irish and Scots dialect for the armpit, originating in the sixteenth century and derived from the Old English *oxta*. So there, oxter has been with us a whole century longer than axilla. I knew I was right.

And while I'm on the subject ...

A is also for axillary node clearance (ANC*)

I had this procedure at the same time as my mastectomy. It involves removing the nodes of the lymphatic system from the armpit. The lymphatic system is part of the immune system and its function seems to be to drain fluid, filter waste and fight infection. The nodes are little bulges situated along this system and on which cancer cells can hitch a ride to the rest of the body.

You'd be forgiven for thinking (as I did before I added the word axilla to my vocabulary) that the doctors are saying *ancillary* node clearance. This would make perfect sense, as it seemed to me if we can do without the damned things, then they were only there in an ancillary or supporting role in the first place. How wrong I was. It is only after you've had your nodes removed that you realise just how crucial they are: you are at lifelong risk of lymphoedema (see page 122), your armpit hurts like hell and the lymphatic system can go into a huff, causing thick, cord-like structures to develop along the affected arm, ouch (see C is for cording).

*ANC. Not to be confused with the African National Congress, which I confess was the first thing I thought of each time someone referred to it. This made me want to smile and raise a fist in solidarity with Nelson Mandela and his chums, but of course I couldn't because my arm hurt so much.

I knew enough from the news and from *ER* to be aware that because cancer can travel to the rest of my body via these lymph nodes, this procedure would be key to my treatment and prognosis. After the operation the nodes would be examined in a laboratory to see how many, if any, were affected. I had seventeen nodes removed from my arm. (Apparently, we all have a different amount, so don't get all competitive if the person in the bed next to you boasts of their twenty-eight nodes compared to your paltry seventeen. I don't know if this has anything to do with the girth of your arm, but I suppose it might. I did ask a few times, but nobody else seemed to find the topic as interesting or vital as I did.)

So I knew node involvement was a big deal, yet even while they were explaining all this to me I found my mind wandering. Node, funny word that. I hadn't said or written the word node since first-form science when the biology master had waxed lyrical about the Node of Ranvier. I have no idea what the Node of Ranvier is, but I never forgot the name. Something to do with sensory neurons, I think. You might have spotted that I have something of an untidy mind, but even for me these lapses were new. Everything the nurses and doctors told me seemed to send me off on a tangent to another place, often to the past. And all these little glimmers of moments from my past comforted and scared me in turn. It was like that cliché that your life flashes before your eyes just before you drown. Only I was drowning in slow motion.

Not having used the word node since I was eleven, I now found I was using it all the time, talking about my nodes as though they were as familiar to me as my eyebrows. These nodes and the complicated transport system they belonged to had never before occupied my thoughts. Now I thought and spoke about them constantly to anyone who cared to listen. Which reminds me – be careful. Don't fall into the trap of becoming a cancer bore. I came dangerously close, so let me take this opportunity to apologise to all my friends. I saw your eyes glaze over, but I kept on regardless. Sorry.

Anyway . . . Axillary Node Clearance. How I came to love those words. Not axillary node biopsy or investigation, but *clearance*. Like slum clearance in the inner cities, paving the way for a bright new future. Clearance meaning riddance. Good riddance.

Waiting for the results of your ANC is nerve wracking and even the most lion-hearted would be forgiven for reaching for the T for tranquillisers. Luckily, you should be too tired from surgery and woozy from the anaesthetic to fully appreciate the strength of your anxiety, but it is still there. And this may sound perverse, but it can still be a positive force.

A is for anger

Get ready to be angry; angry at the cancer, at the medical staff, at your family and friends, at yourself and at all those people who do not have cancer. I have not been this angry since my sister died aged only forty-two from a brain tumour, and I remember it as if it were yesterday. I recall walking out into the street resenting complete strangers – why were they alive when she was dead? – and muttering Shakespeare to myself (I was always inclined to grandiosity):

> Why should a dog, a horse, a rat have life,
> And thou no breath at all?

This anger has come to visit me again. After my diagnosis I saw drunks in the street and thought, Why don't you have cancer? Who would miss you? I came as close as I ever wish to sounding like a bigoted snob, thinking how these drunks and junkies were a drain on society, diverting taxpayers' money from more worthy causes (mine), littering the streets, flaunting their health in my face. Of course, they could have had any number of illnesses for all I knew, but you get the picture. Cancer had turned me from lazy, sometime socialist to half-wit, right-wing harpy. But my darkest hour was yet to come: I stored up my full fury for my son's (absent) father. This much was clear: he should have cancer, not me. He wasn't needed, he wasn't loved, he wasn't even here. I said this out loud to a couple of friends and their reaction was stunned silence and a look that said, 'It's the cancer talking.' And it had to be – because I would not wish this on anyone.

Finally, I was angry with my body, for letting me down.

Don't be surprised if your anger finds odd ways to let itself out. During the first few weeks following my diagnosis I was sometimes overwhelmed by this enormous, impotent rage: a rage that had no language except for the strange noises that came from me. They would start as a low, bovine moan (kind of like a wounded cow), eventually erupting in a desperate howl so loud and so long that I thought once the ground had moved. There should be a new Olympic event – Cry Howling. I would take gold. Thankfully, this period did not last long, but it was not helped by one nurse repeatedly telling me I was taking the diagnosis 'badly'. Although this did give me a new focus for my anger, as I pointed out to her that I'd have to be a complete raving lunatic to take cancer any other way.

A is for affairs (setting them in order)

This is difficult, but once it's done, it's done. Writing a statement setting out my wishes for the care of my ten-year-old son was the hardest thing. As a single parent I felt the onus for me to do this was greater than for others. Imperative, in fact. The trouble was that no matter who I considered as guardian for my son they all had one serious shortcoming: they were not me. But I *had* to do this, so I literally gritted my teeth and sat down at the computer. I was swift and focused. I did not stop until it was done, then I emailed the document to my very sensitive solicitor friend before I had time to doubt. I didn't cry until she emailed me back adding in the words *in the event of my death*. I tasted vomit at the back of my throat. I have never looked at it since.

Of course, I could have waited. No one said I was going to die. I might still be kicking around years from now, but I felt that I couldn't consider undergoing surgery or any other treatment until my son's needs were taken care of. I just couldn't focus until that was sorted. I was also convinced that this would be a lot easier done sooner rather than later and I'm sure I was right. So many people fail to write wills because they imagine they are banging nails in their own coffins, but that simply isn't the case. Writing a will does not precipitate your death, it just makes life less messy. I felt reassured after I'd done it. So what I am saying to you is get this over and done with as quickly as possible and then forget about it.

I also had to make arrangements for my son's immediate care while I was in hospital undergoing surgery. I asked his godmother to come and stay and cleared out the room I used as a study in order to put a bed in it for her. While I was doing this I discovered a mountain of excruciating diaries, letters, bills and photos. Then there were all the notes and plans and dashed dreams that make up most ordinary people's lives, and the thought of anyone accidentally (or deliberately) reading these made me shudder. Imagine the scenario where you've been run over by a bus and your sister or friend has to come and clear out your belongings. Think of it: they might read this stuff. All that embarrassing junk. Think how you would blush (except you wouldn't because you'd be dead, but you know what I mean). A trip to the dump will solve the problem. I cleared out all this detritus from my house, and I can tell you it was one of the most liberating things I've ever done.

Do this early because after your operation you won't be fit enough and later you may lose the impetus. My house and my life are now free from all that STUFF and it feels great. Now I can be run over by that bus with a clear conscience. So there is an up-side to all of this.

A is for admission (to hospital)

Things move quickly when you have cancer. In my mind I was trapped in a kind of suspended animation, unable to get past the words 'It's cancer'. Outside my head though, things moved forward at an alarming rate. Only I wasn't alarmed, I was reassured: the NHS was taking my cancer as seriously as I was.

When the surgeon told me I had cancer and needed surgery I remember thinking it would be ages before I'd be admitted to hospital. I could go home and lick my wounds in secret and not say a word to anyone. Then she told me I'd be admitted within a week or two and I thought the whole idea was preposterous. This was the NHS; did she not know about the waiting lists, the bed shortages? I felt panicked. How fast was this lump inside me growing?

That night I sat on the edge of my son's bed and tried to tell him. I said I might have to have an operation and he squawked '*Surgery!*' like it was the most daring, blasphemous thing he had ever heard. After that I chickened out and couldn't tell him any more, so we settled down to the book we were reading together: *The Adventures of Tom Sawyer*. We reached the chapter where Tom (believed dead) sneaks into church to witness his own funeral and relish how sad all the mourners are. The ten-year-old roared with laughter. I didn't.

I'd left the surgeon saying I'd need some time to prepare my son for the whole experience, then found that I couldn't sit out the wait. I was frantic. I needed this thing cut out of me. I thought of those poor souls who self-harm and visualised myself taking the bread knife to my killer breast. In reality, I knew I'd be leaving the knife work to the experts, so I let the surgeon know that I'd be prepared to come at very short notice after all. And that's what I got: the phone rang at 4.20 p.m. on a Thursday and that same day I was tucked up in my hospital bed, just two weeks to the day since my diagnosis and less than four weeks from the day I'd gone with the lump to the GP. How's that for speed? Let people who criticise the NHS put that in their pipes and smoke it. But even though that time span is so short, it still felt like an eternity. Waiting is one of the worst parts of having cancer. Waiting and worrying. Wondering what your cancer is doing now – is it leaking out into the rest of you like gas from a faulty valve?

I packed in a rush, terrified they'd take the bed from me if I didn't turn up on time. Echoes of the trip to the maternity ward rang in my head, only that time I'd had the bag ready packed in eager anticipation. I tried to stay calm and set about phoning people: my friend who would drive me to the hospital and then move in with my son for the duration; the school, to tell them what was happening and explain there'd be no homework done that night. Like it mattered. I phoned my mother to let her know the time had come. And I talked to my son. I didn't cry. When you are pretending to your child that going in to hospital to have 'cells removed from your armpit' is no big deal, you don't get to cry. But I'm sure he felt my fear. Children do.

Everyone who knows me knows that I talk too much, but all I remember in the car that evening is silence. There were no jokes, no false levity. Then we reached the hospital lifts and saw a sign taped to one of the doors: '2 North has moved to 4 South.' I imagined an entire hospital ward sliding slowly southward like some bizarre form of continental drift. We burst out laughing at the surreal idiocy of it. It was crazy. As crazy as the idea that I had cancer.

I started shivering before we reached the ward, but I didn't falter. A deadening resignation drove me on, like someone going to the gallows: you could try and make a run for it, but what would be the point? They'd get you in the end. So I unpacked my books and bottled water and chocolate and waited. The shivering wouldn't stop; that's what I remember most. Cancer is such a cold place. I got into bed, but I was still cold.

You know that expression 'Youth is wasted on the young'? Well, I have always thought that being off sick is wasted on the sick. And I proved my thesis right that night. There I was, legitimately off work, with nothing to do but lie in bed with a hoard of chocolate and a pile of books I'd not previously had the time to read. Sounds good doesn't it? Unfortunately, the chocolate lost its taste and the books went unread. I couldn't concentrate. Your concentration is one of the first casualties of cancer. You just can't focus to read when you think you are going to die.

I kissed my son goodbye – a small, ordinary kiss on this extraordinary day – and told him not to stay up too late, not to eat too much junk, to brush his teeth, to practise his viola, to catch up on his homework at the weekend. In a sense, none of these things mattered, yet in another sense they mattered even more. Children are conservatives at heart; they like things to be constant. When you take away one of the constants you unsettle them. All the other mundane stuff should remain in place, if only for comfort.

During that week in hospital I agonised over how to tell the ten-year-old the truth about what was happening. I knew I had to, I just didn't know how. Then *Doctor Who* came to the rescue. I asked my friend to buy a DVD of the *Doctor Who* Christmas Special with Kylie Minogue in it. Saint Kylie, back from the dead. I clung to the Kylie Minogue breast cancer recovery story like a child clings to its teddy bear. This *Doctor Who* episode with Kylie in it would allow me a way in to talk about cancer, to show my son that you can have cancer and live another day to sing and pout and maybe even fight some extra-terrestrials too. Poor Kylie – if she only knew the responsibility I was placing on her shoulders. I remember thinking: once I've done the whole Kylie Cancer Hero thing, if she dies, I'll never forgive her.

See also V is for visiting time.

A is for age

Breast cancer makes you young. It's official. Not since my early thirties had anyone referred to me as a younger woman. Turning forty-five is a landmark: I had started to feel middle-aged, but then cancer came along and changed that. In the realm of breast cancer younger may simply be a euphemism for pre-menopausal or it may be to do with the typical age at onset, but all I know is that since my diagnosis doctors and nurses alike have repeatedly referred to me as a 'younger lady'. I am not complaining.

B is for breast

Breast is not a word I often used pre-cancer. It doesn't make me blush, but it does make me a wee bit squeamish. Like a lot of people, I say boobs. I know this is a bit infantile, but the alternative *breasts* has too much of an air of sanctimony about it. It suggests my boobs are something to be revered, respected and taken seriously. Breast has a whispery, sibilant sound to it, whereas boob is more plosive, lip-smacking fun.

Until my diagnosis I'd never really given my less than spec-tacular boobs/breasts much thought. They are fun when having sex, useful when feeding a baby, and essential for making your clothes drape (I've only just discovered this last one). If I were Jordan I would no doubt feel differently, but I am a 34B and will never have career boobs. So when the surgeon told me I had cancer and she would do a total mastectomy I said, 'OK. But can't you take both?' I was told that this was not an option, but despite numerous reassurances I still cannot but think of the remaining boob as the enemy – a time bomb waiting to go off. I kept thinking of Lady Macbeth (told you I was given to grandiosity) and those 'murd'ring ministers' at her breast. And I developed an unhealthy fascination for her 'unsex me here' speech. I know, I know, Lady Macbeth was plotting foul murder, not contemplating a mastectomy, but I couldn't help wondering if having one breast would unsex me.

I do understand that some women would feel traumatised and 'unsexed' by the loss of such a defining part of the anatomy but, on balance, I felt sure that I could live without both my boobs. They were small and past their best. They were, to all intents and purposes, surplus to requirement, and one was potentially killing me.

Before I had time to contemplate the potential psychological impact of being one breast down, the nurse suggested reconstruction and I immediately said yes. My reason was clear: I could not walk around my house with only one boob. Others might tactfully ignore it like the proverbial elephant in the room, but my ten-year-old would surely point out that one of my boobs was missing. A bit like that know-it-all child in 'The Emperor's New Clothes'. A little later, as the operation became more real to me, I started to worry that perhaps I was underestimating the psychological impact of losing one boob – even one I had never much cared for.

So I am not trying to trivialise the experience of having a breast removed. I do know that it is a big deal, and it doesn't matter what age or size you are. Whether you have large or small breasts you will have a lot of adjustments to make, but I think it is worse for large-breasted women because there is such an imbalance. And I also know that being an older woman doesn't mean it will be any less distressing. Why should it? After all, older women have been acquainted with their boobs for a lot longer than the rest of us. The bottom line is this: however distressing you find the idea of a mastectomy you will most likely say, 'Take that boob, take the other one, take my arm too, just let me live.'

See also M is for mastectomy.

B is for bras

If you like lacy, underwired balcony bras you are in for a gruelling time. I suggest you wrap them lovingly in scented tissue paper and hide them at the back of the wardrobe because your breast cancer means that these are a thing of the past. For a while, anyway. In fact, forget ordinary workaday bras too. You may not be wearing regular bras, lacy or otherwise, for quite some time.

The breast care nurses will tell you to buy soft tops with no wiring – a bit like a sports bra, but without the constriction. They will wisely advise you to buy a size bigger than you normally wear. Take this advice; your normal-size bra will be too tight and will cut into your now very delicate skin. I dutifully went out and bought these hideous 'nuns' bras' as I came to think of them, then I put all my old bras into a box in the hope that they'd one day fit me again. (I don't think they ever will.)

Now, I hope this doesn't sound too 'tragedy queen', but when I replay events from that time in my head one of the saddest images I see is of me surreptitiously slipping my bra into a hospital bin after the operation. I remember feeling small and silly and vain and hoped no one had noticed. If my life were a biopic, the director could make much of that small scene as a metaphor for something or other.

See also P is for prosthesis.

B is for breast reconstruction

Brand new boobs, yay! The great thing about breast reconstruction is that you can have it any time, even ten or fifteen years after your mastectomy.

I was lucky enough to have one of the few surgeons in my area who does reconstruction, so the whole process was offered to me and spelled out in eye-watering detail. As I said, my initial reaction to reconstruction was, 'Yep, I'm having that,' but that was when I thought it was as simple as popping in a tooth filling. I thought I'd be ready for my bikini photo shoot in a matter of weeks. Then I found out what was involved.

Reconstructive surgery is not cosmetic surgery: it involves extensive and complicated procedures that move tissue from other parts of the body; sometimes it calls for abdominal surgery too. And, of course, it prolongs the time you are under anaesthetic, means more sites for infections, more wounds, more drains ... And yet I would recommend it, if only because it says: Business As Usual. For me, it was a way of reassuring myself that I had every intention of being around for a very long time and so I'd want both boobs, thank you. However, I was concerned that I would have one brand spanking new boob, all nubile and pert, and a forty-five-year-old one, all wilting and tired. But I needn't have worried. If there is a noticeable disparity between the old and the new your surgeon may offer to reduce, enlarge or lift the other boob so it doesn't look like the ugly step-sister. They can, apparently, even realign your nipples. Mind-boggling.

Another reason I decided to go for reconstruction – and this might sound a bit daft – was because I had this fabulous surgeon whose reputation preceded her, and I thought it an awful waste of her talents if she just did the mastectomy alone. And this will sound even dafter, but I remember thinking she would prefer and even enjoy the task of reconstructing. I felt like I'd be boring her if I had the mastectomy alone, and so she might hand me over to some lesser surgeon. I did say it sounded daft. I am not trying to pretend I had my reconstruction to give my surgeon job satisfaction, but I do remember thinking all of this as they were talking me through the intricacies of the latissimus dorsi flap (which uses muscle from beneath the shoulder blade to form the new breast) and the TRAM flap which uses muscle from the abdomen in the same way. In the end I opted for a tissue expander (an inflatable implant – see page 177) which I considered the least complicated reconstruction available and the only one that did not involve the word 'flap' (unfortunate semantic problem there) and so denied my surgeon that professional challenge anyway.

The breast care nurse was quick to point out to me that breast reconstruction is about symmetry and how you look in a bra. It is not about the naked breast. Even so, it is possible to have nipple reconstruction to improve the appearance of the breast. This can be done by tattooing (sounds excruciating) or by taking skin from a part of the body that most closely resembles the colour and texture of the nipple. The skin is taken from a place I don't want to think about and am too bashful to describe, but if you want to imagine it, then think of the part of your anatomy that has the darkest, purplest skin and you'll get the picture. Ick!

B is for boob club

Yes, I said *boob* club, not book club. Before I went for my surgery the breast care nurse fully prepared me for the experience. I knew about everything from chest drains to how the hospital TV worked. She did an excellent job. She also told me how the women on the ward bonded together to give mutual support and encouragement; a bit like the WI, but without the cakes. So I knew what to expect – but I did not relish the prospect. A disparate group of women would be forced together and we might have nothing in common except our impending or very recent breast surgery. I saw a made-for-TV drama unfolding with little vignettes telling each person's story. (Somebody should write that. I'd watch it.) I imagined us sitting round discussing our stitches and the sizes of our tumours and the whole sorry business, and I thought, No. I will not join your club. I would, I decided, go on the ward and say nothing, or pretend that I was in for an appendectomy or some other non-breast-related procedure.

As it turned out, I was on the ward for less than twenty minutes when a woman called to me from the bed opposite asking what I was in for. I was mortified and angry and I'm sure it showed on my scowling face. I wanted to turn away from her, but I have this problem that means I can't ignore people. If someone asks me something I have to answer them, no matter what. I would be rubbish in Guantanamo; they'd only have to ask me one leading question and I'd 'fess up to anything. And that's what happened on the ward. I wanted to turn from the woman pretending I was hearing impaired, but instead I just stood there like a dummy and told her the truth. Instantly, I was a member of The Boob Club. And I was right; we did discuss stitches and tumour sizes and the amount of fluid in our drains. And the nurse was right; we did support each other.

B is for bravery and battling

How often have you heard the B words? Kylie Minogue is so *brave*. Jade Goody's *battle* against cancer. As if they were standing like Boadicea with sword and shield, fighting a beast. I don't really know what all this battling is about, because for the most part cancer patients are passive: surgery is done *to* you, chemotherapy and radiotherapy too. You don't really have much say in the proceedings. You don't get up and do battle with the linear accelerator in the radiotherapy department; you lie on it like a slab of meat as it battles you.

I suppose what people mean is the mental and emotional effort of trying to keep on top of the situation, and of course, for those whose cancer is advanced, the enormous effort of pushing through what must be intolerable pain. I think walking out in a wig or a bandana certainly takes courage, but unless you are prepared to stay indoors for nearly a whole year, what choice do you have? If you draw the blinds and refuse to come out, your cancer does not go away. If you go under the bedcovers, the cancer goes with you. In the past I looked at cancer patients and asked myself, How do they do that? Now I know. They have no choice.

I am not trying to diminish the experience of others by avoiding the B words. I think of exhausted and sick patients not wanting one more drug or not wanting one more fraction of radiotherapy, getting up out of bed and getting on with it when what they really want to do is lie down. Is that battling? I think of parents putting on a smile for their children and getting up to take them to the park when what they really want to do is cry and sleep, and I suppose that is what they mean by bravery. I see people doing it all around me and some have even said it of me. One friend even suggested that I'd have got more support had I been less brave. I don't know. And what about the people who die? Don't anyone try and tell me they weren't brave enough or didn't fight hard enough. That is just plain insulting.

So bravery and battling remain alien to me. They suggest some kind of fearless, willing action of which I am not capable for the simple reason that I have never been so terrified in all my life. If I could run from this, I would.

C is for clichés and concise conversations

A bizarre and undocumented side effect of cancer is that it makes people talk in clichés. You will lose count of the number of times you hear statements like, 'You're on a roller-coaster of emotions', 'Your health is your wealth', 'Cancer is the great leveller', 'Good health is a lottery'. Don't worry. You'll soon get the hang of it and when someone says to you, 'Rome wasn't built in a day – you have to walk before you can run,' instead of scowling at them, you will find yourself agreeing and mixing metaphors like a veteran. Try 'I can see the silver lining at the end of the tunnel'; or you could simply say, 'It's a small price to pay' (that was my particular favourite when lamenting the missing boob).

Cancer can also adversely affect your ability to converse in words of more than one syllable. The following is the conversation I had on the day I was diagnosed. It was in the school playground and we were waiting for the bell to ring. It was a dark and heavy day, but dry, the worst kind; I could hide behind neither umbrella nor sunglasses. I remember lurking under a tree, hoping that no one would see me. Of course, I was spotted instantly. A friend came up to me and seeing I looked a bit wan and piggy-eyed asked, 'Are you not at work?'

I said, 'No.'

She said, 'Are you sick?'

I said, 'Yeah.'

The bell rang, and as we watched the boys poking around for conkers, she told me that the mother of one of the other children had died the night before.

'How?' I said.

'Breast cancer,' she said.

'Shit,' I said.

C is also for cancer

Obviously. A staggering one in three of us in the UK will get cancer. *One in three*! When I found out this statistic I couldn't stop myself from telling everyone I encountered, and I developed a new and creepy habit of counting round the people in a room to see who number three was. The statistics for breast cancer are just as shocking: nearly 50,000 women diagnosed every year. It is now the most common cancer found in women, and the majority of cases are seen in women over fifty. I was forty-five when I was diagnosed, not that young really, but young enough for me to think that it just bloody well wasn't fair.

Worryingly, no one seems to know what cancer is, or if they do know, they're not letting on. After I had recovered from the initial shock of being told I had cancer, my first impulse was to try and understand not only exactly what it is, but also what causes it. I was told that there aren't causes (see C is for causes), only risk factors, but I wasn't told what these risk factors are.

Obviously, the constraints of time prevent doctors from telling each patient individually what this disease actually is. If they did that, they'd be there all day talking instead of doing, and nobody would want that.

Being told I had cancer was the worst thing that has ever happened to me (there's a surprise) and I needed to understand it. This is tricky: too much information and you might over-load and distress the patient; too little and you might frustrate and distress them. Cancer information seems to range from mind-boggling scientific research studies to the mind-numbing, anodyne 'primer' leaflets they give you at the hospital. Some of the latter left me feeling as ill-informed as the time when, aged eleven, I read a primary school guide to the facts of life. It told me that 'the male and female love cells mingle'. HOW? I wanted to scream. Except I didn't because I didn't want to let on that I didn't know. Some things never change. Now I'm not sure if I should let on that I don't understand cancer, and everyone seems to be assuming that I do. But I am silently screaming, How? And, more importantly, Why?

In desperation I turned to my ten-year-old's science book, according to which we have more than 50 billion cells in our bodies and these are constantly dying and being replenished. The book reminded me that cells reproduce by dividing (oh, how I wished I'd listened when the biology master was bleating on about meiosis and mitosis) and that the process is normally controlled and orderly. I later found out that cancer cells are out of control, as they divide more rapidly than normal cells and so clusters of cells can build up forming a tumour. So at its simplest, I suppose cancer could be described as cell division gone berserk, causing a build-up – like overcrowding. But, of course, it isn't that simple because you can have benign overcrowding and malignant overcrowding. So there must be more to the malignant cells than just the speed at which they divide, right? See how many questions I have? I am now officially fascinated by cell division, and me a literature graduate! (Hooray for cancer; it is helping me bridge the age-old science–arts divide.)

My new-found fascination for all things scientific had me glued to Radio 4's *Start the Week* when they were discussing the secret life of cells. It was riveting stuff. I learned that cells will kill themselves if they are in danger of endangering us. Apparently, most have a 'suicide programme' built in to them to keep us healthy. Not bloody suicidal enough.

Of course, you could have a benign tumour that is relatively harmless unless it's pressing on a vital organ, but most likely if you are reading this, you had a malignant one. And the thing about malignant tumours is not just that they can destroy surrounding tissue, but that they can spread to other parts of the body. By the time I met the oncologist I already knew all about the lymphatic system and how it provided the perfect means for cancer cells to spread, but I was puzzled: the bloodstream seemed to me just as convenient a means of transportation. Why didn't the cancer take this handy and better-known route? (I had this horrible image of the cancer moving malevolently through my blood, spitefully infecting random parts of me along the way.) That might sound like a stupid question to you, and the answer might be obvious to a doctor, but to me, it wasn't. And that is just one of the many clueless questions that can plague the novice cancer patient – and sometimes you feel too stupid to ask. Think back to your school days when the teacher asked that spectacularly silly question, 'Do you understand?' Who among us wanted to admit they didn't? Well I am putting my hand up now. I do not understand.

A diagnosis of cancer is earth shattering and I found that not understanding what was happening made it more so. I know that this will not necessarily be the case for everyone; like I said earlier, I am aware that some people just don't want to know. But whether you are a need-to-know person or a head-in-the-sand person, the single greatest piece of information that you will need to be apprised of is this: a diagnosis of cancer does not have to spell the end. Until I had my diagnosis I didn't actually know of anyone who'd survived breast cancer (apart from Kylie), but I knew plenty who hadn't.

Well the thing is, many people go on to lead long and healthy lives after cancer treatment (according to Macmillan there are 2 million in the UK living with or beyond cancer), but not much is said about them. The trouble seems to be that when someone recovers or is 'cured' of cancer they usually shake the dust from their feet, get back on the bus and we don't hear from them again. And why should we? Their cancer is a thing of the past. They are better. They are getting on with their lives and embracing a new dawn (see what I mean about clichés?), and who can blame them?

C is for conformity

I used to fancy myself as non-conformist. Nothing big or overstated you understand, just low-level stuff, like singing quietly out of tune in the choir to avenge the bully music teacher, or infuriating others by not wanting to marry just because that is what nice girls do. My claim to fame is being voted Head Girl at school, but having the nuns block the vote because I *wasn't right*. They knew I wouldn't toe the line.

Now, however, I desperately want to conform. I want to hear the nurse tell me I am crying the right amount of tears, feeling the right amount of pain, exhibiting the right symptoms. I desperately want to be the good girl and do what is expected of me and know that my cancer is not aberrant. I want to know that they can deal with it.

C is for causes

Doctors talk about risk factors for cancer, not causes. This is unnerving. Cause says to me concrete knowledge and the possibility of cure, whereas 'risk factors' sounds way too nebulous for my liking. Apart from age and genes, about which you can do nothing, these risk factors include health issues such as being overweight, especially after you've had the menopause. NB: I am slim and I have not yet had the menopause.

Hormonal factors are also key. Anything that affects your hormones like HRT and the Pill may increase your risk of breast cancer, as can *not* having babies and not breastfeeding. Guess what? I have always avoided the Pill and I breastfed my baby for ages in the belief that it would protect him from eczema and asthma. I didn't know then that it had the added benefit of protecting against breast cancer. Hurray for breast-feeding! Oh wait, I forgot, he got eczema and asthma, and I got cancer. (Still, I wasn't breastfeeding him merely as a form of medical insurance, so I don't regret it for a minute.) And apparently, starting your periods at a young age also increases the risk of breast cancer. Late developers rejoice. Oh no, hang on again – I was fifteen before my periods started. Not having much luck, am I?

Stress is another factor. This is tricky. You are supposed to remove stress from your life. Well, if you knew how to do that, you wouldn't be stressed in the first place, would you? You'd just see stress coming and take a ring road round it. If only life were that simple. I can't take a diversion around school exams, the economy, the restructuring that is going on at my work. I have to live with it. And here's the rub. Being told you have cancer is stressful. Steer your way round that one.

Finally, lifestyle factors like poor diet and drinking too

much alcohol can also put you at risk. This seems fair to me. How many times have I sanctimoniously looked into other people's shopping trolleys at Tesco and scorned their crisps and white bread and ready meals. I don't eat much junk and I don't smoke, but lest you think I'm some kind of po-faced, born-again health freak, I will admit to really quite liking wine. Recently, Nature has made me cut back by ensuring that I now fall asleep halfway through the second glass (except Cava which wakes me up and makes me love every-one a very great deal). So I'm not an alcoholic, but I do love a drink with my friends. And I am firmly of the belief that having no vices is a vice in itself. Maybe if I just cut back on the Cava . . .

My point is, there are no rules with cancer. It is so damned arbitrary. I bet there is more than one post-menopausal, overweight, Pill-swallowing, HRT-taking, alcohol-swilling, non-breastfeeding, childless woman out there who does not have cancer, and I bet there is more than one saint who does. If you are one such saint, take heart: if you have been doing nothing wrong, you can attract no blame. It is not your fault. And that has got to be good news.

C is for cure

The good news is that cancer is curable, sort of. I think doctors don't like to talk about 'curing' cancer in case they give out false hope. Or perhaps it is that they are being pedants and see cure only as that which they have made well again or a malignant process reversed. They can't really claim they've made something well again if (as in the case of your breast) they've cut it off and destroyed the surrounding area with radiation. However, these measures are a cure of sorts, and if they work, they're good enough for me.

But sometimes doctors do use the 'cure' word. So are they just saying something they think we want to hear, even if it isn't strictly true? Seems unlikely. Good doctors do not make false promises, so if yours talks to you about a 'cure', grab it with both hands and hang on to it.

NB Your chance of a cure is greatly increased the earlier your cancer is detected and treated. So if you are reading this while nursing a lump in your breast, get up and get it checked now.

C is for communication skills (basic level)

This may come as a surprise to some doctors, but I don't usually produce my boobs for people I am not on kissing terms with. Call me old fashioned, but I like a few preliminaries before I take my kit off. So when I meet someone new I like to be fully clothed, otherwise I feel a bit disadvantaged. Many of the doctors I met did take the time to meet me before I got undressed, but not all. And on the occasions when they didn't, I felt a bit affronted. Somebody out there needs to tell doctors that, if time permits, they should step in and say hello before a patient undresses.

C is for consent and choice

If you've ever had an operation you will know that you must sign a consent form before the procedure can go ahead. You will be given a sanitised version of the risks involved but, most likely, you will be too overwrought to clarify the situation. I think I saw lymphoedema listed as one of the possible complications of my operation, but I couldn't swear to it as the whole thing was a bit of a blur. However, I had been well prepared for the operation by the breast care nurse, so I knew what I was letting myself in for and so had no problem signing the consent form.

I think maybe I was spoiled by these brilliant breast care nurses. They took me through my surgical treatment in bald, eye-watering detail. (They leave you in no doubt as to what you are in for.) But they are thin on the ground and they seem to be primarily attached to the surgical team. This means that they are not there to steer you through other treatments like radiotherapy or chemo. Unfortunately for me, this meant that I signed my radiotherapy consent form not fully understanding its contents. I know, I am old enough to know better. I should have asked more questions. I should have taken as long as I liked to read the form, but I felt under pressure. Remember trying to do your school work when the teacher was reading over your shoulder? Impossible. Surely the doctor must have known this. After all, he'd presumably done this countless times, whereas I was a greenhorn. And what if you have literacy problems? It would be like reading Japanese. Backwards. One woman told me her doctor actually read the form to her. I think that is a brilliant idea, but if yours doesn't, let my diffidence be a lesson to you: when they give you a form to sign, read it and question it, no matter how long it takes you.

Greenhorn I may be; complete dimwit I am not. I listen to the news so I know they use ionising radiation in warfare. I remember Chernobyl. And I know why my dentist leaves the room when he takes a two-second X-ray of my gums. So while I was well aware that I was not about to engage in nuclear combat, I did know that radiation was no picnic, and I had begun to worry about swapping my breast cancer for another one, namely, lung cancer. None of the literature I was given made any reference to radiation-therapy-induced cancers, so I asked the doctor about the risk to my lung. He said that *theoretically* it was possible, but the odds were about one in a thousand. And I thought, One in a thousand; not bad, compared with the 1 in 300 risk of other cancers from chemo. Reckon I can just about live with that. Then he added that it was more likely to be skin cancer and handed me the form to sign. Skin cancer, bloody hell! I hadn't even thought of that. I felt a bit stupid and I probably sounded it too. But then, I did say I was a cancer greenhorn.

I think maybe doctors assume consent just because you are sitting before them with that please-save-my-life look on your face, and they see signing the form as a safeguarding formality, and so don't dwell on it too much. In the case of surgery, when you are lying there in your jim-jams waiting, they are probably right to assume consent, but when I turned up at my first oncology and radiotherapy appointments I wasn't consenting to anything. Nor was I refusing anything. I just needed to know and understand what I was consenting to. And I wasn't doubting their expertise either. Asking questions isn't a sign of dissent. It's just a sign that you want to understand.

But even when you do understand you may not feel like you have any choice in the proceedings. One member of staff told me that I did have a choice – that I could say no. And what then? If, like me, you have a young child, your life is not your own to go around rejecting potentially life-saving treatment; you *must* do whatever it is they say it takes. And anyway, how could I, with no medical training or knowledge, decide that I knew better than the doctor who has trained for years and who is trying to cure me? Personally, I never had any intention of rejecting treatment that was offered to me, but what if you did say no – what then? What else is on offer? Nothing, as far as I can see. Your choices are thus: you can choose A or you can choose A. I'll take A thanks. Hobson, I can hear you cheering from your grave.

C is for chemotherapy

I feared this more than any other part of the cancer treatment, partly because I like my head with hair on, and partly because of the very public nature of it. I felt that once I had chemotherapy and was wearing either a wig or bandana the world and his wife would know my business. Nosy-parkers on the school run would cluck together and gasp. Do-gooders would pity me and give me earnest, knowing looks. I couldn't bear it.

I am not going to lie to you; vanity played a large part in my fear of chemotherapy. People were kind and told me it wasn't vanity, and maybe for others it isn't, but for me it was. I knew there were more important things to concern myself about, and if being hairless meant being alive, then so be it. But I was worried sick about what I would look like. Let me paint a picture for you: I wear specs – they are heavy and thick and Nana Mouskouri jokes are rife; I do not have one of those faces that look glorious naked. Without hair I would not look like Sinead O'Connor *circa* 1989; I would look like Harry Hill *circa* 2009.

But mostly, I didn't know how I could prepare my ten-year-old for the experience. I had this preconceived idea that chemo necessarily meant languishing in a well of nausea, weakness and fatigue and I didn't know how my son, being the only other person in the house, could take all that strain. I tested the waters early by saying that some strong medicine might make me tired and make some of my hair come out. He was shocked but told me not to worry; he'd lend me his bandana.

This was all before I discovered what having chemotherapy really entailed. I can honestly say attending that first oncology appointment was one of the most frightening experiences of my life. I think of oncologists as characters in weepy made-for-TV movies. They are the ones that tell you you are going to die. They are usually kind and handsome and a bit syrupy, and somehow we get to feel good even though the beautiful and brave heroine always croaks it in the end. Going to see one made the cancer more scary and chemotherapy was one step closer. I would be the heroine in the weepy, but I wouldn't be beautiful and brave. I'd be wretched and snivelling.

I felt vomit rise at the back of my throat as a young registrar talked me through my eighteen-week chemotherapy plan. He explained that it would be given to me as an outpatient in three-weekly cycles and he described the risks and potential complications involved. I already knew about the fatigue, the nausea and the hair loss, but there was more: blood problems, heart problems, possible life-threatening infections and, worst of all, the risk of other cancers. Suddenly, being a female Harry Hill didn't seem so bad.

I was on the brink of tears throughout this meeting and I think the only thing that stopped me from going in to award-winning weeping was my bewilderment that this doctor seemed to be asking *me* to decide whether or not I should have chemotherapy. (He said I'd have a week or so to make up my mind.) How the heck should I know? I am not a doctor. I asked him what he would do if it were him, but he told me he couldn't answer that question. I couldn't see why not. I wasn't asking him what *I* should do (though it seems to me a fair question for a lay person to ask an expert); I was asking what *he* would do in the same situation. *Tell me what to do*, I wanted to scream. But he wouldn't tell me; the decision was mine.

It was a long meeting, nearly an hour, and as the reality and full horror of chemotherapy became clear to me, the nurse who was with us saw my distress and came and put her arm around me. What strange and wonderful people nurses are that they can comfort complete strangers like that. I'm not sure I could. I felt tears well up in my eyes, but I wasn't blinded. I could see what was happening: setting chemo on the table, making *me* decide, meant that if the treatment nearly killed me, I couldn't blame them; I'd done it to myself. I haven't read *King Richard II* since I was fourteen, when I was so bored that (shame on me) I would sit pencilling in the Os on the page, but these lines came to me from over three decades earlier:

> Mine eyes are full of tears ...
> And yet salt water blinds them not so much
> But they can see ...

See how Shakespeare is always there when I need him? But seriously, I think that maybe both the King and I got it wrong; I think this business of *setting treatment on the table* is really just part of the consent procedure, and rather than divesting themselves of the responsibility for making a decision, the doctors are actually trying to help *us* to make our own informed decisions. But it didn't feel like that at the time. Anyway, I was spared this awful decision in the end because, as it turned out, I didn't have chemotherapy. But that is another story for another day.

C is for counselling

Many cancer charities offer counselling to those affected by cancer. You can refer yourself and the service is free. Brilliant. I would have somewhere to go where I could talk endlessly about my favourite topic: me. Better still, I could just sit there and be as sad or angry or hurt or bloody-minded as I needed without fear of upsetting family or friends. That's the awful thing about cancer: you may be the patient, but you are not the only victim, and if, like me, you have more than your fair share of the guilt gene, you will feel responsible for all the pain your illness has caused. This may mean that you end up managing the flow of information to people, diluting your experiences and pretending everything is fine in case others get upset. And this is wearing, so having somewhere you can go where you don't have to pretend can only be a good thing.

Counselling is also built into the cancer treatment regime. The breast care nurses clearly have a counselling remit and the radiotherapy department has a designated person whose role is information and support (for which read counselling). This is a great idea. After all, this is hopefully as bad as things will ever get for you. You need all the support you can get. Take it.

The problem is that I think counselling can become a sticking plaster that's applied every time things get a little difficult. When I sat gawping at my oncologist, confused by my treatment plan, he suggested counselling. Later, when I became upset (and an eensy bit grumpy) that the consultant in charge of my radiotherapy had not met with me, counselling was suggested. When I burst into tears over my radiotherapy burns and asked to see a dermatologist, counselling was suggested. I know these people are experts, but I am an expert in me and knew how I was feeling. I did not need counselling. I needed information. As if to prove my point, I went independently to a dermatologist about my radiotherapy burns and asked if they would cause skin cancer. The dermatologist understood my concerns, but told me not to worry too much, because if I did get skin cancer, it would be basal cell type and wouldn't kill me. So now I knew. I stopped fretting immediately.

Just in case you're wondering, I'm not one of those people who think counselling is fine *for others*. I did go. I availed myself of the service at my local cancer charity where my counsellor was a fully trained professional who had actually survived cancer herself, so she had empathy in buckets. She was great. Unfortunately, I wasn't. For me, counselling became a repository for all the frustrations I was feeling about my illness and my treatment. I was moaning, and that frustrated me even more, so I stopped going.

I hope I don't sound like I am knocking it. I'm not. Others, no doubt, make more constructive use of the service than I did, and I would urge anyone to make use of this facility. All I am really saying is that counselling should not be used as a get-out clause from answering awkward questions from awkward patients.

I think for me it may have been that I just went at the wrong time; maybe I should have waited until treatment was over before trying to fully process my feelings. I don't know. Anyway, the counsellor I met was down-to-earth and fun and not at all earnest. Best of all, she didn't just sit there and nod, asking, 'And how does that make you feel?' She was actually really supportive. She was especially helpful at the beginning when I had just recently been diagnosed. When I was bawling at her that I didn't want to become a member of the Cancer Club she told me to see it as joining the Survivors' Club. It sounded a bit Disney to me, but it opened a door out of the dark and I am grateful to her.

C is for concentration (or more precisely, lack of it)

This may account for my inability to keep track of my appointments, keys, car park tickets, diary ... Lack of concentration is common when people have suffered illness or trauma, and cancer treatments exacerbate the situation, so it is unlikely that you will escape. Remedial reading material like magazines with lots of big colour pictures can help. Try *Hello!*, *Now*, *OK!* or even *Tatler*. They're usually readily available in hospital/health centre waiting areas, so you won't have to suffer the indignity of actually buying them yourself. The radiotherapy department was especially well stocked, and at that time I became au fait with the affairs of Jennifer Aniston, Fern Britten and her off *The X Factor*.

Loss of concentration came early to me. At the beginning I was simply and understandably preoccupied with my diagnosis, but as time wore on and treatment began, I found it harder and harder to concentrate on any task requiring even the slightest bit of mental effort. Books and newspapers lay unread, conversations were left hanging and TV programmes would take for ever to watch as I would have to keep rewinding in an attempt to follow the simplest of plots.

Perversely, I developed a parallel, one-track mind that could devour whole booklets on the pros and cons of radiotherapy – even the kind I wasn't having (absolutely fascinating), but still could not read more than two short paragraphs of a newspaper article or novel. Even conversations that were not about cancer were difficult to keep track of.

So don't beat yourself up over your lack of concentration. It will get better, *eventually*. In the meantime, keep on trying. Make the effort to read and to listen, and do try not to let your eyes glaze over when it's your friends' turn to talk. There are more things in heaven and earth than cancer, you know.

C is for crying

Talk about Cry Me A River! Never in my life have I ever cried like this. Can you dehydrate from crying? Because after about two weeks of marathon weeping I noticed I was drinking litres more water than usual. I was actually craving the stuff. If I could have drowned the cancer, I'd be cured.

I found I shed three types of tears: angry tears, impotent tears and tears of grief. Grief tears were the worst and the most frequent. I would wake early (around 4 a.m.) and before I had even opened my eyes tears would be falling. These were quiet, shuddering tears choked into my pillow so my son wouldn't hear me from his room. At other times these grief tears would come over me as I watched him doing his homework or playing with his friends or just sitting in front of the

TV and I would have to race from the room. It happened quite a lot at the beginning and when questioned over my red-rimmed eyes, I said that I had developed hay fever. But it doesn't take a genius to see that my grief was simple: cancer could take me away from him.

The impulse to cry can come at any time, but when you have children you control it. And when you are a lone parent like me, you can't just hand the kids over to Daddy and take to your bed with a box of Kleenex. So my crying soon found a rhythm of its own. I would cry during school hours and after bedtime. And not just tears, but enormous ear-splitting screams of despair, like the world had come to an end. Once, returning from the morning school run I only made it to the back door before sliding to the floor, my arms over my head, screaming out in despair. Luckily, the house next to mine was vacant. I was literally bellowing. Sometimes I drove the car out into the country where no one could hear me and roared until I thought my throat would bleed. I only ever did this kind of crying when I was on my own; when I was with friends and family my crying, while still prolific, was a much quieter affair.

I am a great believer in crying and I get cross when I hear of people trying to be in control all the time and denying their emotions. Stoics particularly bug me – except for my mother, the all-time über-stoic. In her I've always found it oddly comforting. Don't get me wrong. I don't want a world where people go around telling me how they feel and blubbing all the time, but some occasions are occasions to cry, and cancer is one of them.

The thing that bothers me about non-criers is that they think they are superior to criers. They see crying as a show of weakness. I, however, am of the opinion that the reverse is true. I think non-criers are too afraid to visit the emotions that will produce an outpouring of tears and so push these feelings away. Criers, on the other hand, have the courage to 'feel and deal' with the emotion and are thus a stronger, healthier bunch of people altogether. There you go: permission to cry.

So crying is a good and healthy response to a cancer diagnosis, and don't let anyone tell you otherwise. And a person's response to your emotion says a lot about them too. The friend who just holds your hand and lets you cry is a blessing; but don't be too harsh on friends who find all this emotion hard – they are suffering too. Medical professionals, however, are another matter. One nurse seemed to be of the opinion that all this emotion was pathological. She tried to medicalise (is there such a word?) my emotions: 'You're taking this badly,' she kept saying. 'Go and see your GP. To tide you over.' I couldn't really see the point in going to my doctor unless it was to have someone different to cry to, but I did it anyway. The GP knew why I had been sent and offered me tranquillisers and sleeping tablets and anti-depressants. I am not against medication, but this felt like adding insult to injury. So when I was admitted to hospital and another nurse said softly to me, 'It's important to cry, you know,' I could have kissed her. Honestly, if you can't cry at a time like this, when can you?

Crying is part of cancer. But you can't go around weeping and wailing all the time. You still have to live in the world, so you will have to control your emotions, like it or not. It is bad form to cry over the fruit and veg at your local supermarket; it is helping no one if you blub it all out to the man in the post office. There is a time and a place. But *do* make that time to cry and don't let anyone make you feel that your tears are not valid.

C is for consultant

When you have cancer your consultant, a mere mortal, takes on epic proportions. This is the person in whose hands you lay your life. This is the person you pin all your hopes on, and it is to them that you offer your silent prayer: *save me*.

No pressure, then.

But first, some consultant-related etiquette. Consultant surgeons should be addressed as Miss, Mrs or Mr – not Doctor. You might as well start off on the right foot: don't want to upset the person with the knife. The breast care nurse told me about the Mr/Miss thing at our first meeting and I remember thinking it a daft piece of information, but filed it just the same, in case my surgeon proved title-conscious.

I was assigned to three consultants: one for surgery, one for drug therapies (chemo/hormonal) and one for radiotherapy. I believe these last two are oncologists, one medical and one clinical, but for simplicity I will refer to them as the consultant oncologist and the radiotherapy consultant respectively.

Consultants are the highest up the chain of command that you are likely to meet; they get paid more than the other doctors, have more expertise and experience and they're thinner on the ground, so you cannot always expect to have a lengthy appointment with yours. A swift glance around the crowded waiting rooms at most clinics will give you an idea of the workload these people have. Make the most of your slot with the consultant.

I am told that the consultant oncologist does, in fact, oversee all my treatment, but I haven't been able to confirm this. And I have heard some people say that they only felt really cared for when they met with their oncologist; they felt able to forge a relationship with this person and felt looked after. Unfortunately, I never had that experience and, I'm not going to lie, it was a disappointment. (Although much later I did meet a female oncologist who impressed me and with whom I think I could have had such a relationship.)

Meanwhile, in radiotherapy, I never got to meet my consultant. I did ask, but it never happened. Generally, I consider philosophy to be a little irritating and more than a little beyond my grasp (it occurs to me that the second point probably explains the first), but recent experience has caused my mind to wander to the work of the French philosopher and semiotician Roland Barthes. He wrote some Clever Dick stuff about how certain sections of society (the disabled for instance) are not visible in the media, and coined the phrase *absent presence* to describe the phenomenon. They are there, but we are not permitted to see them. Blimey! Just like my radiotherapy consultant. So philosophy does have its uses. The only solution I can think of for the absent-presence problem is to make a big stink and insist on your right to see your consultant. I tried this and failed. (The philosophers probably have a phrase for that too.)

My surgical consultation was another matter entirely. Right from the start I knew that I was in expert hands, and I can honestly say that with the surgical team looking after me I felt safe. Cynics might mock, but the notion of safety is central to an experience like this. The consultant surgeon and her team did such a good job of it that they, and the building that housed them (which was separate from the other treatment areas), became for me a totem for all that is good in the NHS.

The consultant surgeon was efficient, attentive, informative and confident, and clearly took great pride in her work. Reassuringly, she guided her registrars closely, and while they might not have liked that at times (I'm guessing), it paid off because they too were all excellent, though I'm sure she can't take all the credit.

My first impulse after meeting the surgeon was to find out more about her. She had the ability to be businesslike and compassionate at the same time, and I liked the way she got straight to the point, but I was still uneasy. I needn't have worried. Preliminary investigations told me that my surgeon was 'f**king brilliant', no less. I told my son (no, not the f**king part, just the bit about her being brilliant) and he said, 'She better be.'

In addition to her reputation for being brilliant, she had a Nordic-sounding name, and a nice line in monogrammed scrubs. My mind filled with vague remembered stories of Norse gods and goddesses and my imagination ran wild. Cool, my very own avenging angel. I pictured her slicing off my breast to the strains of Wagner's 'Ride of the Valkyries', triumphantly saving me from the clutches of death. It is a mark of how much she impressed me that I was able to be so frivolous with my fantasies. Had I been worried, I'd have imagined her lopping off the wrong boob while I lay paralysed, yet – by some freak of anaesthesia – conscious and able to hear the Wagner for myself.

And the hours these people work. My consultant surgeon

was in that hospital morning, noon and night, and weekends too. My operation was scheduled for a Friday, but was cancelled at the last minute because of a gunshot victim who took ages to fix. I thought of thugs I'd never know planning a shooting and butterflies flapping their wings in the Amazon: chaos theory. I cursed the thugs and assumed – it being the weekend – that I would be sent home to await another date while my surgeon went off to the golf course. And why shouldn't she? It was the weekend, after all; everyone is entitled to time off. But no, I was taken the very next morning. How's that for service!

And yes, I do know that the NHS has its detractors but fair's fair – when it's good, it is excellent.

NB Since beginning my treatment I have also been treated by excellent bowel and gynae surgeons (both men, both consultants), so no conclusions can be drawn about gender here.

C is for checking

It really was a small miracle that I found my lump when I did. I had more or less given up checking my breasts and had justified this cavalier attitude to my health by repeatedly joking that lump hunting was pointless. I had so many lumps and bumps that it was like feeling blindfold for a particular pea in a sack full of them. So when my test came back positive for cancer I was filled with self-loathing. How could I have let this happen? I felt ashamed, like someone caught not brushing their teeth. And I was doubly ashamed because I have a young son I need to be with; the least I could do was check for lumps every few weeks.

But if you have had a similar experience, don't beat yourself up about it. I've learned this will do you no good whatsoever. Put it behind you, but do start checking your breasts regularly. The nurses will give you guidance on how best to do this or you can go online to any of the major cancer charities for advice. And don't become complacent just because you have been scheduled for yearly mammograms following your diagnosis. This doesn't let you off the hook. Tumours can develop in between scans, so it is up to you to check and check and check, and report any changes however small, and however much you fear sounding like a total neurotic.

C is for cloth ears and clumsy questions

Have you noticed how some people seem to suffer from Cloth Ear? You ask them a question and they respond with silence or a confounding and bizarre non-sequitur that conveniently brings the conversation down another, safer path. Come on, you must know someone – an elderly relative, your boss, your partner maybe? You know the kind of thing I mean:

> You: Can I have a pay rise?
> Boss: Did you see where I put my stapler?

Well, when you have cancer the problem gets worse. Either that or my communication skills hit a new low, because my questions kept getting lost in translation:

> Me: Doctor, Doctor, are there any alternatives to Tamoxifen?
> Doctor: Have you considered counselling?

I know I've already made the point about counselling (see page 47), but I do have a serious opinion to share about communication.

My problem is that I am so afraid of sounding bolshie and confrontational, of being defined as the 'problem patient', that my queries sometimes sound like apologies not questions, and so go unheard. Doctors, for their part, may wish to protect patients whom they consider are not ready to learn the full extent of their condition, so they might glide over the difficult bits. If you're not careful, you could end up partnered in an exhausting and fruitless shadow dance.

This is tricky. I presume doctors are under obligation to tell patients something about their illness and treatment, even if the patients don't want to hear it. And the trouble is that some people really don't want to know, and some of us really do. I know one woman who told her doctors to just get on with it and tell her nothing, and I suppose that's fine for her, but I am one of those people who likes knowing things. Especially things about me. So patients' differing preferences in terms of information (or lack of it) must put doctors under added stress; but if we don't ask, or they can't give the curious enough information, we could end up in the arms of Doctor Internet. A dangerous liaison indeed. At a time like this Google is just as likely to become your worst enemy as your best friend.

My old history teacher (I had a crush on him and so I always listened attentively) told us that knowledge without understanding is a dangerous thing. I believed him. Still do. When I was first diagnosed I could have become an internet junkie, filling up on case studies and statistics, symptoms and survival rates, but I thought, No – I will not do that. And if I am honest, I am irked by people who talk like experts just because they read something on Wikipedia. (You can just hear the consultant, can't you: 'Hmm, read that on the internet, did you dear?')

You see, I am an old-fashioned respecter of expertise. I reckon these doctors have studied long and hard to get where they are today and I think we should show them due respect. Unless, of course, they refuse to answer any of your questions and treat you like a numpty. Then you might turn to the internet.*

Of course, no website can properly take the place of patient–doctor talk, especially when that talk is good. Let me give you an example: after being on Tamoxifen for a while, I went to my GP suffering from repeated, annoying urinary tract infections. Instead of saying, 'That's probably the Tamoxifen' (or, God forbid, suggesting counselling), he actually gave me (unprompted) a potted biology lesson about how the bladder and uterus form in the unborn and explained why the drug might, therefore, affect all of my plumbing. Fascinating. I kept getting the urinary tract infections, but it kind of took the sting out of the situation, if you know what I mean. Because now it all made sense.

C is for cording

A few days after breast surgery my armpit/axilla/oxter started to ache. I reached in and found a mass of hard, tight, rope-like

---

*Tread carefully in cyberspace; it is full of wormholes and wackos. (See I is for internet junkie; and also P is for probably.)

structures that had grown there like a forbidden forest. Two days later I could barely move my arm and the ropes were now visible down the entire length of my arm. This could not be normal. I didn't even bother with the doctor or the breast care nurses, but went straight to the physiotherapist I'd met on the ward. Hadn't she told me to report any odd changes? Didn't ropes in your armpit constitute odd? Would she think I had lost the plot completely? 'Ropes in your armpit dear, really?' Would she refer me on to psychiatry?

'That will be cording,' she told me down the phone, very matter of fact. 'Come in and see me tomorrow.' And there began months of painful physiotherapy. Really painful. Chinese torture painful. I actually screamed out loud once. But one by one she snapped the cords (not ropes) and restored my arm to working order.

A standard joke among doctors and nurses is to call physiotherapists physio-terrorists (I bet they get really fed up with that one), and after you've had cording, you'll know why. In my case it was all worth it though. Not only was my physio expert at administering eye-watering massages, she was nice and friendly and full of information and, best of all, averse to bullshit. I am sure I was sent cording by my guardian angel so that I could meet this physio and she could keep my spirits up and explain what was happening to me. After the initial meetings with the breast care nurses, she was the single greatest source of information and guidance I received. Thank

God I didn't get some tight-lipped listener who nodded earnestly when I cried. Thank God she did not suggest counselling.

I can find no definitive description of cording; all references to it are prefaced with words like *it seems to be* or *it is thought to be*. Well ... it is thought to be a hardening/scarring/congestion of the lymph vessels after ANC. But don't expect anyone outside post-operative breast surgery to have a blind clue what it is. GPs won't know and doctors from other disciplines will be equally unaware of it. As for how it feels – the only way I can explain it is as though all the ligaments and tendons in your arm have been drawn tight and are too short for your arm to function properly. When mine was at its worst it felt like my arm would break if I tried to straighten it. At one point I was in such pain I actually fantasised about this. But they don't offer arm breaking on the NHS, so I had to content myself with the slow, excruciating burn of the massage.

For many women cording is, apparently, so painful that they cannot bear to have physiotherapy. I do understand this, but if you develop it, do try and put yourself through treatment. A good physio will know when to stop and when to push on. And you never know, you might get some peace of mind at the same time.

C is for complementary and alternative therapies

Know this: conventional doctors do not like unconventional therapies. I sat among a group of breast cancer patients one day and listened to countless stories of doctors warning against other therapies. I have met no doctors who speak out against *complementary* therapy, but I'm sure that no doctor will sanction you replacing conventional cancer medicine with *alternative* remedies.

I have to admit that when I am surrounded by people who embrace alternative therapies I feel a bit boring, something of a fuddy duddy – like a conservative at a rave. It is not for me. But I will say this: I bet any of us, doctors included, would willingly eat grass with a knife and fork if we thought it would save us. Lots of people dabble in alternative therapies at some time or other, even if it is only a cup of herbal tea and a lie-down instead of reaching for painkillers when they have a headache. I do it myself. But when it comes to the big things I am still willing to place my faith in conventional medicine and doctors. I would have to be extremely well informed and feel extremely confident in that information before I could disregard what the doctor was saying. However, I do understand that if you are facing your second round of cancer treatment, you may well feel disillusioned with conventional medicine and wish to try the alternatives. I might feel the same in that situation. I think where cancer is concerned it is less about being alternative and more about being desperate. But what I am saying is, you can't expect that your doctor will sanction it. It goes against their training.

My experience is that while doctors may frown upon or even condemn alternative therapies, most will encourage you to avail yourself of complementary ones. These focus on your emotional well-being – something doctors may have neither the time, expertise or patience to deal with. And this is where the cancer charities come into play. Many offer a range of complementary therapies designed to help you back to health or help you deal with ill health, whichever is appropriate. They include exercise classes, art and writing therapies, relaxation and meditation, and reflexology among others. All of these are expertly carried out and you can try as many as you like for free. Yes, free. Go along and explore these services, especially as your treatment comes to an end. At that time you can start to feel cast aside, like yesterday's news, and these programmes can help you through that tricky phase. And don't let your prejudices stand in the way. Even if you do not think your feet are the windows to the sole, sorry I mean soul, try reflexology anyway: at worst, you will get a nice-smelling massage while listening to some soothing music.

I joined a yoga class at which the very lovely and bendy instructor contorted herself into various positions and tried to make us do the same. There was a great emphasis on relaxation and it was all very gentle and safe, while still giving my weak arm a really good workout. I would recommend yoga to anyone, but I never got that glow the others had. While they were connecting with their inner selves, I was busy wondering what to have for tea that night or worrying that I'd left the cooker on. I just couldn't get in the 'zone'.

I also joined a relaxation class after one therapist suggested I wasn't ready for reflexology as I was too tense and needed to relax (I thought that was the point!); I watched as others surrendered themselves to statements like 'Love holds the planets in orbit', and felt like an infidel in a mosque for thinking that, really, it was boring old gravity.

But these therapies do work for many people, and while some of those I tried were not for me (I was too ticklish in the end for reflexology and too distrustful for relaxation/visualisation), I can't praise them enough. I often found myself watching enviously as others emerged truly glowing with contentment, leaving me behind – the wallflower at the dance.

C is for charities

There are a lot of good charity organisations out there doing brilliant work for cancer, and they need to be applauded. On the day I was diagnosed, the breast care nurse gave me a leaflet about the Macmillan centre and I thought, What did she give me this for? Am I dying? Isn't that what Macmillan is for? Well, yes it is; and no it isn't.

Macmillan offers support (practical, emotional, financial) to *anyone* affected by cancer. It is run in partnership with other major cancer charities (so you can get introduced to those too). I found this was excellent because I made contact with my local charity and reaped the rewards. All of the staff I met in both charities were kind and tactful. And when I eventually plucked up the courage to walk through one charity's doors I saw that it was not populated by the morose, wasted souls I had expected. It was populated by people who – like me – were determined to get better.

I found the staff there amazing, the surroundings pleasant, the services offered brilliant. I tried yoga, art therapy and reflexology (with varying degrees of success). And I got enormous help from their Citizens' Advice Bureau (especially good if, like me, you are form-phobic, as they can help you fill in those daunting health questionnaires and benefit forms). And it was *all* free.

Next time you pass a collection tin for a cancer charity, drop in a few coins. Or better still, set up a direct debit.

C is for complaining

At some time or other every woman (and one man) I know has looked into the mirror at the hairdresser's and cringed: they have been given a bob when they asked for a Mohican. And what do they do? Do they complain? No. They smile at the hairdresser, say, 'Thank you, that's great' and leave, choking back the tears and telling themselves it looks nice from the back.

When it comes to complaining, my experience of doctors and hairdressers differs little. Needless to say, the consequences of being given the equivalent of a wrong 'do' by a doctor could be catastrophic and much more distressing, but my reaction in this circumstance would be no different. Fool that I am, I would thank them, then go home to weep. I do not complain because I don't want to make a fuss; I don't want to be seen as a whinger; I don't want to get anyone into trouble (especially a rookie) and, wait for it, I don't want to hurt their feelings. Nor do I want to prejudice my future care. The doctor and I would be forced to meet again and I would never know if he has performed the medical equivalent of spitting in my soup, but would always be wary.

I think the problem with complaining is that people confuse it with moaning. Moaning and complaining are two very different activities. Moaning is when you repeatedly drone on about what went wrong, but do nothing constructive about it; complaining is when you take control.

Complaining takes courage. It is pointing out that something went wrong and needs to be put right. Think of it as being like reporting a fault. OK, it's too late to remedy the situation for yourself, but think of all the women coming after you. And although you will be so physically and mentally tired from treatment that you will not have the strength to sit down and pen a coherent letter, you can jot down dates and problems and then set them aside for a few months until you are strong enough to write one. Your complaint should still be valid up to six months after the incident took place and sometimes this can be extended.

I think complaining is tricky because a badly handled complaint could actually cause you some stress, but if you do have a genuine grievance and don't complain, the danger is that you will nurse it into a monster. Airing grievances can be cathartic. William Blake – artist, poet and sometimes madman – got it right when he expressed the view that if you communicate your feelings, you resolve things for the better. Keep it to yourself and woe betide you:

> I was angry with my friend;
> I told my wrath, my wrath did end.
> I was angry with my foe:
> I told it not, my wrath did grow.
>> From 'A Poison Tree'

Or, put more prosaically: better out than in. So if you don't want to end up watering your complaint night and morning with your tears and growing yourself a great big poison tree, speak out. Write that letter and do us all a favour. (See also Resources, page 213, for organisations that can help you with filing a complaint; best not to go it alone.)

NB The flip side of this is that you should give praise where praise is due. Do it. It is not hard to send a card or small gift of thanks to the staff who have done a good job. And while you're at it, don't just remember the medical staff. Spare a thought for that nice woman who works on the enquiry desk or the secretary who rearranged that appointment for you.

D is for diagnosis

It can take as little as a few hours to be diagnosed with breast cancer. I went to a specialist one-stop clinic that provides an amazing and efficient service and promises your results the same day. It's something to see the work they do there.

I never believed for one moment that I would have cancer. Not once. Not even when, after the mammogram, I had an ultrasound scan followed by an FNA (fine needle aspiration). The fine needle aspiration is a short procedure where they insert a (not so fine) needle into your breast and draw out cells from the lump. It hurts a bit, but it's over fairly quickly. If you have an FNA, do not panic. It does not mean you have cancer. It is often used to drain benign cysts. I had cysts. I knew that. They'd told me so the year before, so while I was nervous about all the poking and prodding, I wasn't really worried.

Then, just as I was leaving the mammography suite a member of staff held my gaze for too long, and I knew. And at that moment everything slowed down and all around the sounds of the busy hospital wing came to me muffled, as if heard underwater. Soon I was being led down a corridor where a nurse glanced at me, a fraction of a second only, then looked at the registrar who was walking alongside me and I saw that they both knew what was coming. I was ushered into a small strategically placed room (you don't have to walk back through the other patients) and once inside, the slow motion/underwater sound trick stopped.

There were three people in the room: the consultant, a nurse and a registrar, and I thought, It does not take three people to tell you you are fine. They sat me in front of the consultant who said cancer. As plain as that. As if cancer was something you said every day. She was very matter of fact and offered no promises. I remember pulling back from her and repeating the word *No* over and over, like a toddler who has just discovered the ability to assert himself. But no amount of saying no would change the diagnosis. I also cried big, fat tears like a toddler. Infantilising business this cancer.

I remember being shocked by the surgeon's directness, and then grateful. Try not to be upset if you feel your surgeon is being blunt with you. Had mine been less clear, I might have left thinking I had something *like* cancer, but not quite cancer – some pre-cancerous nearly-nearly disease. I could have told myself so many lies.

Then it hit me that they were wrong. I pointed out to my surgeon that I am a lone parent and I have a young son to look after: ergo, I could not possibly have cancer. But she remained convinced. Then I remembered my mother: eighty-four years of age and having already buried one daughter. How could I ever tell her? I was sandwiched between two generations of people I could not possibly tell this awful thing to.

When the surgeon had finished explaining what treatment I would need, the two doctors left, but the nurse stayed with me to mop up my tears and prepare me for the next stage. She was the 'Breast Care Nurse'. Funny, I was crying a good bit and feeling seriously sorry for myself, but I still found myself thinking, I bet they don't refer to the Testicle Care Nurse when it's men's bits they're dealing with. Anyway, this nurse must have done this a lot because she was a mine of information and she really did an excellent job of preparing me for what lay ahead. But she had an incredibly ponderous way of communicating which I assumed she'd perfected at some kind of 'talking-to-the-distressed' workshop where they teach you to talk very firmly and v-e-r-y s-l-o-w-l-y. Presumably, we need it. And obviously it works because I remember almost every word she said to me (and it is well known that patients supposedly recall only about half of what they are told in consultations).

In 'real life', the nurse probably talks at normal speed and is really just very good at her job. And God! What a job she had. At one point she had to push me off her as I had literally thrown myself on her and was bawling into her crotch, like a hammy actor in an awful soap. I do freely admit to being an emotional person, but I can honestly say that is the first (and I hope the last) time that I have ever physically thrown myself on a complete stranger. I remember thinking, God! What am I doing? – but doing it anyway.

They advise you to bring someone with you to these meetings and maybe that is the reason why. If you need a crotch to cry into, bring your own. I, however, had come alone, and although the nurse kept urging me to ring someone to come and get me and be with me, I couldn't see the point in that. Friends were at work or on holiday; and what good would it do to ruin someone else's day? But the nurse was persistent and I didn't want to look like Norman No Mates, so I texted a friend to phone me, knowing that she was forty miles away and that she would not read the text for hours anyway. My advice to everyone now however is: take someone with you even if, like me, you think you are going to be fine. Because eventually, four hours after I'd arrived, I left the hospital as I had come – alone; and I have never felt so lonely in all my life.

D is for disclosure

Not long before my diagnosis my son and I were listening to a comedy show on the radio where the comedian was poking fun at mobile phone etiquette. He pointed out that the word cancer is now included in predictive 'speed' text programmes and hilariously sketched out a scenario whereby you informed loved ones of your diagnosis via text message:

I've got cancer :(

My son and I hooted with laughter and went about making the dinner. Only weeks later I received my diagnosis and was faced with the problem of who to tell and how. I checked my mobile; it does have cancer on predictive text.

My first instinct was to tell no one. Medical folk take the stance that openness and honesty are best when dealing with your cancer diagnosis and treatment. They will urge you to be frank and, at any rate, not to lie. I wasn't so sure. Lying

suddenly seemed like a virtue. I imagined this elaborate subterfuge: I would tell people I was having my appendix out and
pretend that nothing much was wrong. I would bankrupt
myself getting the most expensive wig money could buy. I
would tell work I wanted a sabbatical. I would not go out
unless I absolutely, positively had to … Clearly, I was
deranged. Do not follow my example; no good will come of
it. You will become isolated and lonely and lost, and you'll
still have cancer.

If I heard about someone who did as I'd planned, I would
have no sympathy for them. I would think them misguided
at best, a sanctimonious martyr at worst. But I wasn't trying
to be a martyr. I just could not think how on earth I could
tell my son and my mother that I had this killer inside me.
(At that stage I assumed cancer meant death.) So for three
long days following diagnosis I holed myself up inside my
house and told no one. Perversely, during that time I often
thought to stop the postman or the meter man or some
other passer-by and tell them instead that I had cancer and
let them walk away with it and never come back. I felt I
could tell people who didn't really exist in my life, but that
once I'd told friends and family it would be like letting the
cancer in, making it real. Well, here is the news: it already is
real and you need to tell people. You cannot do this cancer
thing alone.

Eventually, I accepted that I had to say cancer out loud, but

I would not tell my son. It was different for us: a lone parent and an only child. How could I let him carry that burden? This became my constant refrain – 'It's different for us.' And so it is. None of the literature I read seemed to realise that single-parent families even exist. None of the practitioners I met knew how to respond when I kept up my chorus, 'It's different for us.'

I was given a book to help my son come to terms with cancer treatment. It had lovely illustrations of an ever-so-sweet family getting to grips with cancer, and I could identify with none of it. It only served to ram home my point about cosy stereotypes my son would never relate to: the bungling but caring dad; the pretty yet plain mum (who didn't look too bad in a bandana, actually); the two cute bewildered children; the pet; the charmingly dishevelled house; the youthful grandparents. None of this was us. I live with my son in a city miles away from any relations, and even if Granny and Grandad (both octogenarian diabetics) did live next door, we'd more likely be popping in to check their insulin levels to make sure they make it to their next birthdays. There would be no trips with Grandad to the park to fly kites, no jaunty little picnics in the spring. I put the book away. It was different for us.

So no one could offer me any help and I had no answers. All I knew was that I was right: it is different for us and for that reason honesty is even more important. I do think there is a case for not telling very young children if your prognosis is good and you are expected to make a full recovery, but otherwise you will have to tell them and help them and that is a tough job. Most of the lone parents (of only children) that I know have really close relationships with their children, much more so than those in conventional two-parent families where the tie is diluted by numbers. I have always had a very open relationship with my son and apart from a few memorable exceptions (see H is for honesty) I do not knowingly lie to him. So I told him the truth, but I did it slowly, by degrees, and I have to admit that I did not get it right at first.

Apart from the betrayal aspect of lying to your children, there is also the fact that it is really quite stupid. No matter how careful you are, if your child has normal hearing and normal intelligence, chances are they will overhear someone say the word mastectomy or cancer or chemotherapy or radiotherapy. All they have to do is look the word up and your goose will be cooked. Better to hear it from you than from Wikipedia. And then there are the countless leaflets you are given – one for just about every aspect of your treatment (which is just as well considering the taciturnity of some doctors; I now have two folders full of the things, covering everything from the initial 'welcome pack' the breast care nurse gave me on day one to the last leaflet I received from the Cancer Centre on how to cope with lymphoedema). Each one carries the word cancer on it, so you will have to find somewhere very secure to store these and be disciplined about keeping them concealed if you don't want your children to see them. Imagine if they stumbled on that material by accident. There'd be hell to pay.

Some women told me their reaction to the diagnosis was to tell everyone they met. I totally understand this. And I do have experience of doing something similar. Although initially, I told only a select group of friends, about five months into my treatment I entered a new but short-lived phase, telling three people in the space of a week before going silent again. These were people who did not need to know and who rarely saw me, so what possessed me? Was it Glasnost or verbal incontinence? I can just hear the amateur psychologists out there saying that they might not need to know, but I needed to tell. Maybe. Does it matter? Perhaps *saying* 'cancer' is the first step to dealing with it, whether you whisper it or shout it out. You know what they say: to slay the beast, first you must say its name.

See also W is for wildfire.

D is for drugs

No, not the kind they have at raves. I mean prescription drugs – the ones the doctors give you to take the sting out of life. And cancer. My GP offered me the works, if I wanted them – tranquillisers, anti-depressants and sleeping tablets. I didn't take the tranquillisers. I thought it unwise as they might actually diminish my ability to deal with stress and could be addictive. Slippery slope. I looked into my crystal ball and saw myself taking diazepam every time the car wouldn't start or I ran out of Bran Flakes. I agreed to a prescription for anti-depressants but never actually took the pills. I just kept them in a drawer by my bed for their placebo effect. Somehow, just knowing they were there meant never having to take them. Makes no sense I know, but it worked. Besides, I wasn't depressed. I was sad. Sadness is not an illness; it is a rational response to sorrowful events.

The sleeping tablets were a different matter. Two weeks into my cancer diagnosis and I was already seriously sleep deprived. I could not keep this up. If I didn't get a night's sleep soon I would go out of my mind. When my GP suggested them I thought of Shakespeare again, *Othello* this time (I did warn you):

> Not poppy, nor mandragora,
> Nor all the drowsy syrups of the world,
> Shall ever medicine [me] to that sweet sleep
> which [I] owed'st yesterday.

Seriously, I never knew Shakespeare was lurking in my

head like this, but you'll be relieved to know that I didn't actually say this to the doctor. I said thank you and took the prescription. I took the sleeping tablets and the result was not much sleep, stinking hangover, monumental migraine and a mouth that felt as though I had been sucking on old socks. It took me a while to figure out that the sleeping tablets were causing all of these symptoms though (not the brightest, I know), after which I stopped taking them. I am not suggesting that you should eschew all and any drugs designed to help with your equilibrium. If you need it, take it. You wouldn't have your teeth out without anaesthetic so why suffer this difficult time unaided, right? I am just saying that for me at that time it wasn't right. I may feel differently next week or next year.

Part of the problem with drugs is that they actually cause problems. Anti-depressants* take roughly three weeks to kick in, tranquillisers are addictive and sleeping tablets give you a hangover. Imagine the poor ten-year-old having to deal with that train wreck. No, cancer was enough. Those women whose husband or partner or family were there to pick up the pieces could have the drugs. I couldn't afford to.

*Be careful: some anti-depressants reportedly interfere with the working of the cancer drug Tamoxifen. Double-check with your doctor and oncologist.

D is for denial

I have heard it said that denial is part of the cancer patient's profile. Guess what? I fit the profile.

On the day I was diagnosed the doctor advised me to inform my son's school. This is good advice. Take it. Children need adults looking out for them at a time like this. After several days of Cry Howling (see A is for anger) I dutifully made my way to my son's teacher. I did not have an appointment, but as I had cried all that day I figured I was too wrung out to blub in front of him and so seized my chance. We went into a small office. Neither of us sat down and I just said in a very whispery voice, 'I have cancer' – as bald as that. I remember having difficulty keeping eye contact with him. I felt sorry for him because he didn't know how to deal with this and was obviously terrified that I would start to cry. He hadn't trained for this. Neither had I.

We agreed that he would keep a discreet eye on my son, then said goodbye. I remember him saying, 'I'm sorry for your news', and I thought, That's what they say at funerals: 'I'm sorry for your trouble.' The next thing I remember, I was running. I was out of breath by the time I reached my car where the ten-year-old was waiting for me, bored, having run on ahead. My heart was pounding in a *Looney Tune* way and I remember looking down to see if it was pushing out through the wall of my chest, cartoon-style. I headed home, but the traffic was bad; Chelsea tractors and trucks the size of small houses bringing schoolchildren home sat bumper to bumper, and the journey took ages. Ages enough for a strange thing to happen in my brain. I managed to convince myself that I had lied to the teacher; that I had gone to him all washed out and red-eyed and told the whopper of the century. I supposed he was already with the headmaster and they were discussing how best to deal with (and protect children from) lying, hypochondriac, Munchausen, psycho-mummies who were trying desperately to find ways around the 11+ exam. I began to sweat.

That's when I had this crazy thought: I could abandon the car, go back to the school and tell the teacher it was a mistake before he had a chance to speak to the headmaster. And then the sane part of me chimed in pointing out that the teacher would think me deranged. Perhaps I was. I stayed in the car (thank you God) and somehow made it home.

I made a plan. I would ring the breast care nurse and tell her what had happened and she would write a letter explaining that there had been a mix-up. Even as I took the nurse's card from my purse and dialled her number it did not occur to me that I had it for a reason. Her answering machine kicked in (thank you God again) and I didn't leave a message; I just hung up and slumped to the floor as it dawned on me what was happening.

I took out the information pack the nurse had given me

and read the storybook entitled *Mummy's Lump*, designed to help me talk to my son. I puzzled over the leaflet on breast reconstruction. I had this stuff for a reason. I hadn't lied. This was real.

Now that is what I call denial.

D is for depression

Everyone assumes me to be depressed. Instead of being the hidden beast that embarrasses everyone, when you have cancer, depression becomes socially acceptable. More acceptable than the cancer itself. What a pity then that I'm not depressed. I wouldn't have to lie about it and paint a fake smile on my face.

I know why they think I am depressed: they are confusing sadness and fear with depression. I have never, ever felt this sad, and I am *literally* scared for my life, but I am not depressed. Depression is a feeling of removal and a removal of feeling, of being devoid of emotion, vacant. I am overwhelmed by emotion; it is choking me, erupting from me, drowning me. But I am not depressed. Not yet.

What is depressing is the tendency for some people (and most medical folk) to pathologise normal human emotion in this way. Crying when you have been given a diagnosis of cancer is not a sign of mental illness. It is a sign of good sense. People should learn to tell the difference between the two.

See also C is for crying.

D is for disability

This is a tricky one. Without a white stick or a wheelchair you may find the term disability erroneous and misplaced when applied to you, but don't go all D for denial over it. While not actually a disability, cancer is covered by the Disability Discrimination Act and it offers you protection and help in the workplace, which is good to know. I spent a lot of time in ignorance, fearing I might lose my job if I took the recommended six to twelve months off. If only I'd known.

You may also be entitled to DLA (Disability Living Allowance). You know, that benefit the tabloids tell us is a honeypot for dole scroungers and ne'er-do-wells suffering from the fabled bad back? If you've always worked to earn a crust, you may find it difficult to make the leap to apply for DLA. Don't let pride stand in the way. Fill in the forms (the Macmillan Centre can assist) and take all the help you can get.

The Macmillan Centre can also advise you on other benefits you might be entitled to, like help with rent and rates, tax credits, travel and health costs. Or they can advise on grants and loans. The thing about having cancer is that it can actually cost you money and not just in lost earnings. You may have to buy equipment or a wig and you will have to travel frequently to hospital. And remember, the children still need to be fed. You will have to start tightening your belt when you are knocked back to half pay and if the judo class or swimming lessons have to go, then cancer is doubly ruining your child's life. They will feel miserable and you will feel guilty. So take what you can. You didn't make this cancer up, you know.

D is for discharge (from hospital)

The length of time you spend in hospital for your mastectomy varies. I was in for a week, but another woman who was admitted on the same day went home before me. In any case, you don't get to go home until all your drains are clear and have been removed. Until then, you go rattling around the ward with your drain bottles (see page 88) gathered up in a plastic bag. Not chic. Being a one-boobed bag lady brought out a side of me I didn't know existed. I even asked a friend to bring me in a 'good-quality' plastic bag – one that wouldn't rattle so much and would look nice. Think of Margot from the 1970s comedy *The Good Life* snootily scorning a super-market plastic bag in favour of a Harrods holdall and you'll get the picture. The things you learn about yourself when you have cancer!

Assuming everything else is fine, once your drains have gone, you can go. You'd think this would be good news, but as discharge day drew near I felt panicked. I was terrified. I didn't admit this to anyone because unless you've been in the situation you won't understand it. You will never comprehend why a perfectly normal person would want to stay in a dormitory full of people who are snoring and crying and waking you up all the time. A place full of foul smells and weak tea; a place where they serve you dinner at five o' clock in the afternoon. And yet if they'd have let me, I'd have stayed.

Going home seemed impossible. I'd never manage. I couldn't get out of bed and make breakfast or wash dishes or check homework, or know if my wound was OK. I couldn't *cope*. If you live alone, take my advice: find someone to stay with you. I can't believe I actually thought I could do this on my own. Thankfully for me, the friend who had stayed with my son agreed to stay another week and so going home wasn't quite so daunting in the end. Even so, I still didn't think I could cope.

I wonder if medical staff realise just how scary going home really is. I wonder if they know that the fear isn't just about the practical, but the psychological too. I felt that once I'd left the security of the hospital ward I would be on my own with the cancer again. That week in hospital was seven slack days during which I could abdicate responsibility for my own health. Once home, I'd have to step up and take control again. How could I possibly do that?

D is for drains

A funny thing happened to me on the way to the loo ... I was clutching my plastic bag of drains at the time and whichever way I twisted round to lock the toilet door, one of them came loose from its collection bottle. I stared, horrified, as bloody fluid spewed everywhere – on my slippers, my PJs, the walls. I thought I'd better stop it before the place looked like the shower scene from *Psycho*, and tried to grab hold of the tubes, but they kept escaping me as though they had a life of their own. I was like a cartoon dog chasing its tail and I started to panic at the sight of all the blood spilling from me.

I considered pushing the alarm button for a nurse to come and help me before all my precious blood leaked out on to the floor, but then I remembered the drains were *meant* to be draining fluid *from* me *into* the bottles. So I wasn't bleeding to death, just making an awful bloody mess.

I grabbed the tubes and shoved them back in the bottles. Simple as that. Simple me. I blame the anaesthetic for addling my brain.

D is for diary

If you don't already have a diary, buy one. Cancer brings a whole new structure to your life and a whole raft of appointments and consultations you couldn't possibly remember unaided. On 17 September my diary stopped detailing meetings and lectures and training days, instead showing hospital appointments with surgeons, oncologists, radiotherapists, physiotherapists and X-rays, scans, reviews ... I couldn't keep up. My brain had turned to mush and now I had a new career as personal assistant to a sick person.

At first, I tried scribbling the dates in code (to protect the ten-year-old) on the kitchen wall planner, but the code was so cryptic I hadn't a clue what it meant. Try figuring out what *Ref.Texp2* means a week after you've written it and see how far you get. For the longest time I thought my radiotherapy appointments (RT) were simply reminders to buy the *Radio Times*. Far easier to keep a diary and leave the hieroglyphics to someone else.

(You will also find this diary essential if you are given

hormonal therapy – to keep track of your now possibly erratic menstrual cycle, see under H.)

D is also for death

But I am not going there.

E is for epiphany

I feel short-changed. All around me cancer patients are having epiphanies. The scales are falling from their eyes and they are finally seeing what life is really all about. They are getting their priorities right, throwing off their shackles, putting love first. I envy them; they look born again. I can't join in though because I always knew what mattered, to me, anyway. I always put love first. Unfortunately, it didn't always put me first.

I also always lived for the moment and as a consequence my pension plan wouldn't even feed my cat, if I had one. I've never understood people who don't worry about the nature and quality of their daily existence. I suppose they are too caught up in the act of doing, of working and making money, of bringing up their families to give it thought. These are the people who wait till middle age before asking, *What's it all about?* These are the people who don't get depressed or hung up on existentialism. Lucky them. Twice lucky, because now they are having their epiphanies. I want one too.

E is for epidemic

When I first stepped through the revolving doors of the cancer centre at my local hospital I was immediately struck by the hordes of people milling around. They couldn't all have cancer, could they? All these people: it was like an epidemic.

I went to hide out in the centre's café, but it was so busy I couldn't get a seat. I lurked in a corner studiously avoiding eye contact with everyone in the building, even the receptionist. I wanted people to think I was just a visitor or that I worked there. I was afraid if they looked in my eyes they would know I had cancer. Weird, I know.

A word of advice: subterfuge is futile. Don't even try it. The number of bald heads and bandanas quickly gives the game away. Because of the vast numbers of patients being attended to every day at cancer hospitals, some have a system whereby you check in at reception and are given a disc which vibrates

and buzzes when it's your turn. This should alert you immediately to expect a long wait, but at least you can amble down
to the shop while you are waiting or wander the corridors
playing guess the artist (an interesting collection of artwork
adorns the walls). This disc system works really well and you
quickly get used to it, but I have to admit that I couldn't help
thinking of lepers ringing bells to warn others of their
approach. Still, at least it means you can always slip out to the
toilets for a good cry without fear of missing your slot.

On that first day, lurking in the foyer of the cancer centre
I remember thinking if the shopping centres were as busy as
this there would be no recession. I looked at the staff and
thought: your job is safe. The government should forget
about retraining big city bankers and stockbroker types for
the teaching profession, I thought; there is a future to be had
in cancer.

And you know what? All those people, all that waiting
around and, refreshingly, I never once heard anyone make a
fuss. Maybe like me, they were tossing the figures over in
their minds: one in three people in the UK will get cancer.
One in three. Or maybe they were thinking that there is
safety in numbers. Maybe we should take comfort from
knowing that we are not alone. This is a big problem. They
will fix it. Won't they?

E is for euphemisms

Euphemisms are the mild, innocuous terms we use to disguise unpleasant or offensive things. They make the bad things seem more palatable, less troublesome. According to the dictionary, the word euphemism comes from the Greek *euphemismos* – to speak words of good omen. *Euphemismos*, sounds like a spell, doesn't it? If only ...

Think of all the euphemisms for dying and death. Few people just up and die, they 'pass away', 'go west', 'join the choir invisible', 'kick the bucket', 'croak it' or simply are 'at rest'. And the number of euphemisms for illness is just as impressive: take problems with your 'waterworks' or having 'the trots' for starters. And should you suffer a complete mental breakdown and walk out naked into the street, handing out daisies to strangers, you won't be clinically insane, you'd be 'a sandwich short of a picnic'.

Sometimes we even whisper the euphemism, as if saying it out loud is an invitation to the disease to take hold. This is because euphemisms are rooted in superstition. I've never been superstitious. Until now. If I say the word cancer out loud, will it bring me bad luck?

So euphemisms are a good thing, right? They spare our feelings. They let us down gently. But what happens when they go wrong? A child told that a dead person is only sleeping may develop a fear of bedtime. A cancer patient who is told they have 'a mass' or 'a growth' or 'a cell cluster' may leave the consulting room with no clue as to what is actually wrong with them. And what about 'The C-word' or the term 'The Big C' used to describe cancer? I swear, as a young child seeing this phrase mouthed silently struck more fear into my heart than the word cancer shouted aloud ever could. So you see, sometimes euphemisms can be counterproductive and even dangerous. I believe doctors are now instructed to avoid euphemisms and tell us how it really is. My surgeon certainly did and I am grateful to her for that, though it was a body blow at the time.

Euphemisms are especially dangerous when dealing with children. I should know. I fell foul of them when I tried to talk to my son about my treatment. I think of myself as all grown-up and broad-minded and hip, but what did I do? I told him I was having an operation to remove some *cells from my armpit*. I know, hypocrite, hypocrite and thrice hypocrite, but it was all I could manage at the time. After my little chat, the poor child had no clue as to what was going on and I had subsequently to revisit 'telling' him several times, to hammer the message home. I had succeeded only in confusing the boy, and when he eventually understood he said, 'No harm to you Mum, but you did a rubbish job of telling me that.'

So euphemisms, while generally well-meaning, can be misleading and damaging and are best avoided. I am all against them.

Or am I?

When I was having my cancer treatment one of the doctors made me laugh by speculating about how the hospital unit I was being treated in got its name. I imagined a sitcom boardroom filled with trustees and executives and market researchers and PR people. They'd been given an important brief: a new and exciting central facility catering for all types of cancer has been built. It houses state-of-the-art equipment and a highly skilled workforce. It is bright and spacious. It has a garden with a water feature. It needs a name.

I amused myself imagining the discussions they might have had, the disputes and debates, the names they might have discarded. They might have chosen a name deriving from a townland or former landmark that paid due deference to the past and allowed patients to enter the building without the taxi driver dropping them off knowing what was wrong. But oh no! What do the collective great minds in the boardroom come up with? *Cancer Centre.*

All across the UK, health authorities are abandoning naming hospital facilities after saints and eminent physicians in favour of saying it 'like it really is'. I blame Oprah and that Dr Phil of hers. Now, in order to get treatment, every patient, young and old alike, has to walk under a banner that points the finger and screams *Cancer*!

I like to think of myself as being fairly broad-minded, so

I hate to be the one criticising this particular brand of openness as it is no doubt designed to demystify and destigmatise the disease. The problem is I don't think it does. I feel no less frightened by cancer because I see its name writ large. It just delivers a slap in the face every time I pass through that door. So maybe euphemisms do have a place, sometimes.

If you are still not convinced, let me put it this way: imagine a building with a huge, shiny sign above its door saying *Erectile Dysfunction Unit*. Need I say more?

PS Someone recently told me that the patients themselves helped choose the name 'Cancer Centre'. Reckon they embraced H for honesty too wholeheartedly.

F is for five years

Cancer doctors talk about five-year survival rates. When I first heard this I nearly choked. What good was five years to me? I needed twenty-five, and some more. But don't panic when you hear about five-year survival rates. This doesn't mean that you are only being given five years to live. However, it also doesn't mean that if you are still alive after five years you are free of cancer *for ever*. There are no for evers in cancer.

As far as I can tell, all the five-year thing means is that the research studies that track cancer patients extend over the five years following first treatment. After that they do not report on these people. The figures simply show the percentage of people still alive after five years and tell nothing of what happens to them in subsequent years, even if they go on to live healthily for decades.

Try not to get too hung up on statistics and studies, particularly if they are bad. Remember, your cancer is unique to you and the statistics you are reading may not take into account the specifics of your case. And don't forget, research studies take time to complete, so the information you are reading could already be out of date. If you are going to go down this route, always check the date of the study you are reading. If it is several years old, it can't take into account advances – like a new drug or even the availability of that drug – made in the past year or two and these might be significant.

So don't get too down if you don't like what you see. Wait for the next study or, better still, avoid them altogether.

See also S is for statistics.

F is for fatigue

I am tired of telling people that I am tired and they are tired of hearing it. But I am, even now, months after the treatment has ended.

Fatigue in cancer is much talked about. You will be given fatigue leaflets and fatigue books and fatigue diaries. They even hold fatigue workshops.

As I see it, the trouble with fatigue isn't that it is so debilitating; it's that it isn't cured by sleeping, and it can affect you for months and even years (apparently), long after treatment has finished. The only up-side that I can think of here is that doctors and nurses are not afraid to talk about it, and so you know exactly what to expect. I got to the point where I expected to be sleepwalking twenty-four/seven and was over the moon when that wasn't the case. They had prepared me for the worst and anything less was a gift. I felt charmed. See, there is a strong argument for telling patients how it really might be.

The thing about fatigue is that it is *so boring*. You feel like a sloth and you look a mess because even combing your hair (if you're lucky enough to have any) seems like a monumental task. You will have to find a way through this, making adjustments now and well into the future, so start getting used to the idea. I am currently considering being a good girl and going to bed before 11 p.m. to see if that helps, but the idea frightens me, making me a child again – like being in one of those cheesy, teen, body-swap movies and having to sit my O Level maths all over again. Maybe I'll try exercise instead and see if that helps.

See also Z is for ZZZzs.

F is for flight socks

They make you wear compression stockings for the duration of your stay in hospital. These are more or less the same as the socks worn by passengers on long-haul flights to protect against thrombosis and swelling. They are white, knee-length, open-toed monstrosities. A bit like a geriatric version of the knee socks you wore as a child. Except that you are not a child and you look ridiculous. Find the silver lining: you will not have to shave your legs for the duration.

G is for grief

The emotion I most experienced on being diagnosed with cancer was grief. It was like a death had occurred. I was grieving for the life I might never have, all those things I had yet to do. Things at home, things at work, holiday things. As time passed these concerns fell away, but I found myself still grieving. For one reason only: my son. This made me want to hug him and cry and eat chocolate with him and watch *Lassie* movies late into the night. We didn't though. We just went on as if nothing was wrong, doing boring homework, practising boring scales, tea at teatime, bed at bedtime. Business as usual. Don't hurt your children with your grief.

I believe that grief can be a positive force and should be felt, but if it's very fierce, do it in private or with grown-ups, and when it is done put it away. This might sound a bit New Age, but you could try visualising your grief on a shelf at the back of the wardrobe or in a drawer you don't use much. I keep mine in a box with the bras I no longer wear. Obviously, this is a bit simplistic and I think it only works if you have expressed, not repressed, your grief. But by doing this you are not denying your grief, but neither are you allowing it to consume you. And you have to do *something*, otherwise your grief could become cheapened by overexposure and spill over into self-pity, and you know nobody likes a whinger. (You'll know you've hit self-pity when you start crying about all the bad things that happened in your past and how you have no luck and blah blah blah.) Pitying oneself and grieving are two very different activities. Allow yourself to grieve. Then stop.

See also S is for self-pity.

G is for Goody (Jade)

Poor Jade Goody is dead. Only twenty-seven and with two small boys. It's heartbreaking. The BBC News tells me you either liked Jade Goody or you didn't. I didn't, and I have to admit I was upset seeing her die so publicly like that, especially when I was trying to convince my son (and myself) that cancer doesn't have to mean the end. One cancer patient I met who was also uncomfortable with it said to me, 'Sure she's only going through the same as the rest of us.' (Except, of course, that she is dead and we are still alive.)

And you can't help wondering if things could have been different: if only she'd gone for a smear sooner; if only treatment had started earlier; if only . . .

But as much as I was initially repulsed to see Jade Goody dying on TV, I think I do understand it a bit. Maybe she was simply saying this: 'I am on TV, therefore I am alive.' And who could fault her for wanting that? And in a way she is still 'alive', because here I am talking about her.

When she died it was a mark of the huge impact she had made that the Prime Minister stood up and eulogised her. But what about the rest of us? The news tells me that Britain lags behind other major European countries for cancer survival rates. Why doesn't the government put its money where its mouth is and find out why?

NB Don't neglect your cervical smear. Jade Goody RIP.

G is for guilt

Let me explain about my relationship with guilt: it is stead-
fast, robust and enduring. It will not go away. If I pass a *Big
Issue* seller and don't give them any money, I will be racked
with guilt for a week. I have even been known to drive back
to the scene of my neglect and give money to a seller I'd previously ignored. Then, if I take the magazine, I feel guilty as
they need it more than I do – because if I don't take it, they
could, in effect, sell it twice. The ten-year-old tells me this is
what I am meant to do. But if I don't take the magazine I feel
guilty that I will seem a smug, patronising, middle-class do-
gooder, polishing my halo in public. So you see, I take my
guilt very seriously.

Cancer opens up a whole new dimension of guilt. Layer
upon layer of it. Guilt over how you got the disease in the first
place, guilt over the strain you are placing on friends and family,
about leaving work colleagues in the lurch, about not being so
much fun with your child. It really is one great big guiltfest.

I will never forget the day I told my mother I had cancer.
The guilt was impressive even by my standards. I was terrified
and approached her like a naughty child who had done a bad

thing. I thought she might be cross with me*: firstly, for having cancer, and secondly, for getting found out. I felt *so* guilty: had I done this to myself? Had I allowed work to stress me out too much? Had I drunk too much alcohol, eaten the wrong food, slept the wrong sleep? Getting cancer was so totally irresponsible, especially as I have a young son to take care of. My mother would point out that he depended entirely on me and I would be consumed. How could I have let this happen?

Find a paper bag and breathe into it. A lot of cancer guilt is irrational and pointless, but not all. If you are guilty of not checking your breasts, start now. If you are guilty of smoking, get help to give up. If you eat junk, try to improve your diet. If you're a lush, cut back. Otherwise, stop feeling guilty. It is a waste of time and energy. Most likely the cancer is not your fault. Save your energy for getting better. You'll need it.

H is for honesty

What is it with people and honesty all of a sudden?

Now that I had cancer I was supposed to be an open book, it seemed. But why? And why was everyone pretending that

---

*Of course my mother wasn't cross; she just swallowed hard.

we don't lie to our children? Had they forgotten all about Santa and the Tooth Fairy? Apparently, I needed to tell my son that I would be going to radiotherapy because I would be leaving the house every day. Hello? I already did leave the house every day. I wouldn't tell him if I were leaving the house to have sex with someone I met on the internet; I'd tell him I was popping out to the shops. Apparently, I also had to be honest about the medication I'd be taking because it could make me feel sick and tired. But if I were taking medication for gonorrhoea, guess what? I wouldn't tell him. I'd say I was feeling a bit off and probably lie that the tablets were vitamins.

I did eventually swallow the honesty pill though and told my son the truth. I wasn't one hundred per cent convinced at the time, but I did it anyway. Now, I really, truly and absolutely believe this was the right thing to do. Although when a friend asked me what she would tell *her* son I wanted to scream, 'Tell him I'm having a vaginoplasty' (not that I need one, you understand). Why on earth would her son need to know anything other than that I was feeling a bit unwell at that time? Honest to God, honesty gone mad.

H is for help

Being brave? Soldiering on? Think twice. My advice is to slow down, ask for and take all the help you can get. Especially at the start and at difficult times during treatment.

I tried to limit the amount of help my friends gave me because I was afraid they might get compassion fatigue or that it would be too much for them. (They didn't and it wasn't.) I, however, quickly became exhausted from pretending I could do things that were too much for me. You will need help with shopping, cooking, cleaning, laundry, ironing, childcare and transport (as you may not be able to drive for a while). You will also need emotional support. That's a lot of help. Ask and let people know.

After surgery my right arm (my dominant one) was weak and sore and the cording (see page 62) made it more so. I knew I couldn't possibly cope at home on my own. I couldn't successfully lift a kettle with the affected arm, so draining a pot of spuds was a non-starter. Later, the cording meant I couldn't even raise my arm far enough to take a cup down from a shelf. Was I really expected to cope on my own? Did they think I was making up the bit about being a lone parent? Was I the only patient who had no family living within spitting distance? I didn't want to put all the burden on my friends, so I asked to speak to the hospital social worker and I knew immediately that help was almost non-existent.

However, there was one service that seemed hopeful, promising practical help on my return home from hospital. Perfect. I agreed to try it and a few days after I was discharged a nice woman came and offered to help me get dressed. She also offered to fetch some light shopping for me, but no, she could not help me with the cooking, nor the housework, nor help me put on a wash, nor peg it out. If I could not even wash or dress myself how the heck was I expected to run my home, feed and look after myself and a ten-year-old?

I was left with no choice. I swallowed my pride and asked my friends. And I have never regretted it. If it hadn't been for the friend who stayed a week after I left hospital, the ten-year-old and I would've lived on badly buttered toast for the duration.

H is for hypochondria

I am now a fully paid-up, lifetime member of the hypochondriacs' club. For every twinge and ache I feel I think, *cancer*. I am particularly concerned about uterine cancer (see H is for hormonal therapy).

My GP tells me these feelings are normal and shows no sign of tedium when I tell her of a new worry. She tells me that for the next twenty years they too will think cancer at each of my aches and pains. Twenty years. I like the way she said that. So ordinary. So matter of fact. I have become used to how reductive cancer is: I used to have vague ambitions for work and for travel. I haven't seen the pyramids or the Great Wall of China yet. Suddenly, these don't matter any more and my ambition is diminished: I want only to be alive.

So I will continue to take each and every ache to the doctor. Do the same and don't apologise, until one day, eventually, just being alive will no longer be enough.

H is for hope

You must keep believing that tomorrow or next week or next year will bring some breakthrough in cancer treatment, even if your doctors stubbornly refuse to give you hope. They don't want to give false hopes and they don't want to be sued when it backfires. And that's fine for them, but you must never stop hoping. Hope makes you human. Hope keeps you alive.

H is for hormonal therapy

Some cancers thrive on hormones. If, for example, they tell you your cancer is PR positive, it means that the cancer cells thrive on the hormone progesterone. ER positive means that cancer cell growth is stimulated by the oestrogen produced in your body. The solution seems obvious: stop the oestrogen supply. Apparently, the cancer drug Tamoxifen does just this by stopping the oestrogen reaching the cancer cells, and I'm told it is very successful in reducing breast cancer recurrence.

Of course, any drug that interferes with your hormones will not be without drawbacks. I was wary. I immediately asked the nurse about side effects and she explained that Tamoxifen is taken for a five-year period during which time I could expect to experience an array of symptoms from hot flushes to weight gain. The list of side effects is so impressive that it really is not a good idea to read them all. Just wait and see what happens to you. And be prepared for a delayed reaction: one woman I know didn't start getting hot flushes until she had been on the drug for a year. The breast care nurse gave me a leaflet on Tamoxifen and said that as well as menopause-like symptoms there were other, rarer, side effects that I should be aware of. Such as? Such as failing vision, hirsutism and a deepening of the singing voice. I pictured myself a blind and bearded baritone. Move over Andrea Bocelli – a star is born. We had a laugh and moved on to the next symptom, uterine cancer. I stopped laughing. That's the problem with cancer treatments from chemo to hormonal to radiation therapy – they can all potentially cause new cancers to develop. Add *double-edged sword* to your list of clichés.

I was very worried about uterine cancer and wanted to know what screening is offered. The answer is none. Screening is not routinely offered to women taking Tamoxifen. You have to present with symptoms. Symptoms like irregular bleeding. Well guess what? Tamoxifen causes irregularities in your menstrual cycle. How on earth are you to tell the difference between one type of irregular bleeding and another? My periods have gone haywire, is this safe or unsafe irregular bleeding? God, I wish I'd married a doctor.

The first thing to do here is to keep a strict record of the bleeding in your diary. If, after a while, you are convinced that your cycle is well and truly 'up the left' go and see your GP and ask to see a specialist. I waited five months because I felt the doctors wouldn't take me seriously until I'd given the drug a chance. But I don't think you should leave it so long if you are having major irregularities. Remember, the main person looking out for you at this point is you.

This is a lot to worry about. But you will have to establish a hierarchy of worries because, presumably, you are not going to get uterine cancer after swallowing one or two pills, so push it down the list. That will give you time to focus on the more imminent problems of nausea (I felt sea sick for about six weeks), fatigue and the dreaded menopausal symptoms. What larks, a chemically induced false menopause. (Daft word menopause, isn't a pause meant to be a *temporary* cessation?)

Anyway, I envisaged myself tired, crabby, flushed and sweating, plagued by near psychotic mood swings and reckoned I needed to prepare the ten-year-old. I told him that I would be taking some tablets for a while that might make me a bit tired and crabby. After a marked pause he looked up at me and smiled; I smiled back, and we said in unison, 'No change there then.'

H is for Herceptin

I did not need the breast cancer drug Herceptin, but I feel I have to mention it because it has been so widely reported in the media that it is practically a household name. Even those who know next to nothing of cancer have heard of Herceptin. This is due to the high-profile case of Ann Marie Rogers who successfully took her health authority to court in 2006 for denying her access to the drug on financial grounds. As a result of her efforts the drug was funded for widespread use on the NHS and all newly diagnosed women are now routinely tested to see if the drug is appropriate for them. So if you are getting Herceptin, it seems it is largely down to one woman's efforts. What an achievement. That woman certainly had something to be proud of.

On day one, the breast care nurse told me that I would

have a Herceptin profile done and I eagerly awaited its outcome, Herceptin being generally regarded by lay people as a wonder drug which I therefore, of course, wanted. I didn't get it and wondered why. I kept on asking about it, but each time was told the results weren't back yet. Eventually, I discovered that I had tested HER2 negative. Herceptin would have been useless as it works by targeting the HER2 protein that fuels some cancers. And in any case, it is usually given alongside chemotherapy.

It took a long time for me to find out all this, and all the while I was thinking they'd forgotten about me or that legislation concerning the drug had not yet reached my health authority. In fact, I think they weren't telling me about it because I wasn't going to need it. That seems fair enough; these doctors are under pressure and barely have time to talk about the treatments you are having, never mind those you are not. So I think if you want to know about all the types of treatment available (and not available) to you, you will have to ask. Time is tight; they won't volunteer the information.

I is for internet junkie

When one of the registrars told me that I would need Tamoxifen, I asked him if there were any alternatives that had fewer side effects (I fancied neither beard nor menopause – see page 107) and he said, 'Well, you might read that on the internet, but really there isn't.'

This, before I had even dared to log on! I was fuming. Of course, the effect was to send me dashing off into cyberspace. Now I *had* to know. And so I learned from Doctor Internet that Tamoxifen is appropriate in my case because I am pre-menopausal, that alternative drugs are usually only available and effective for older (i.e. menopausal) women, and that Tamoxifen is tried and tested and the first drug of choice for my type of oestrogen-related cancer.

I suppose I should thank that doctor for (unwittingly) forcing me to log on because until then I had been studiously avoiding my computer, eyeing it nervously and treating it like the enemy. Instead of being a useful tool for keeping in touch with people via email, my computer had become a potential harbinger of doom and scary statistics, mortality rates and horror stories. Or so I thought. When I eventually logged on I found that cancer websites aren't really scary at all. They are anaesthetised places with lots of white space where information is measured out in carefully worded portions. They go easy on you.

That said, my advice to you is, do not become an internet junkie. It is not healthy to sit researching cancer all day and the chances are that a lot of what you read will be incomprehensible unless you have a medical degree. And remember, any wacko or mischief maker can post an entry on the internet, and many do. Apparently, it has been reported on the internet that David Beckham was an eighteenth-century Chinese goalkeeper, that Robbie Williams eats pet hamsters for a lark and that Plato was an ancient Hawaiian surfer. See what I mean?

But let's face it, this is the digital age and the internet is the place where most of us get most of our information, so I'd recommend that you go to the websites of established organisations. There are loads of good cancer charity websites out there. I had to go no further than the Macmillan/cancerbackup site, and I wish I had known about it sooner. It offers a comprehensive range of information that has been very carefully worded so as not to distress. Still, although websites like this are written for the lay person and are excellent, nothing beats a proper doctor–patient talk.

A lot of people use message boards to communicate and gain information about cancer. These can be a great source of support, especially if you live in a rural area where services are few, but I would be very wary of depending on 'chat' as a source of information. There are a lot of us out there trying to make sense of what our doctors are and aren't telling us, and while these platforms provide help and encouragement, you still have to exercise some caution. It is at times like this that unhelpful comparisons can be made. Another person's cancer and circumstances will be different from yours, so you can't go thinking you should be treated the same. You can sensibly use the internet to help fill in the blanks your doctor has left, but you'll still need proper help to understand all of this. Make friends with your GP or breast care nurse.

Fascinating Internet Junkie fact: cancer is the second most-searched topic on the internet after pornography. I know this because *Newsnight* told me so.

I is for infection

Cancer is a hypochondriac's dream come true. For the rest of us it is a bloody nightmare. Everything makes you sick, even the cures. Even seemingly minor infections can become worrying very quickly.

Those having chemotherapy will be warned to be extra careful not to expose themselves to unnecessary dangers (like visiting someone you know to be sick). My friend's father became gravely ill following an infection contracted while undergoing chemotherapy, and my cousin worried us all when she was taken into hospital with a fever during her chemo. She is fine now, and thankfully patients suffering serious infections seem to be in the minority, but you need to be so careful. Radiotherapy also carries risks, so you will need to be vigilant.

After axillary node clearance (see page 10) the lymphatic system is unable to fight infection effectively. For this reason you will be told to avoid any activity that could endanger that area, like a cut, graze or burn. I almost bit a phlebotomist who tried to draw blood from my bad arm. She looked upset, but I felt she should have known. Surely my notes said *right-sided* mastectomy and ANC. At the risk of repeating myself, you are the one who has to be on the lookout, and that can be difficult when you're punch drunk from an anaesthetic or bawling your eyes out at some new development.

Following ANC and radiotherapy the risk of limb swelling (lymphoedema) is high, and so they will advise you not to lift hot items from the oven with your affected arm, not to carry heavy shopping with it and not to sport your shoulder bag on that side. They will also tell you not to shave that armpit (in the interests of symmetry I let both sides grow out, ick), not to use scissors to cut your nails and to be careful of knife blades when washing up. Yet, nonsensically, they will tell you to 'pin' your soft prosthesis to your underwear. Sure, if you want an arm the size of a seal pup. If a nick on your finger sustained from nail scissors can cause lymphoedema, then surely being stabbed by a safety pin in the fresh-from-surgery breast will do the same, only quicker. Seems logical to me, but if that's not the case I need an explanation as to why not. They will also tell you to be careful when swimming in the sea and in a swimming pool; be cautious when exercising; don't expose the affected arm to the sun. Hmm ... I'm thinking of patenting the first long-sleeved, one-armed bikini.

Honestly, you begin to feel like one of those cranks who invent things to worry about, but apparently you really do have to be this careful. However, I think you also have to be realistic and pragmatic about this. One member of staff told me not to spend time at the beach or let that arm see the sun. What kind of summer holiday would I have standing in my burka watching the ten-year-old have a splash? So I will swim, but I will be careful to use factor 50 and to cover up quickly afterwards. I want to live in the world, not on the sidelines.

Bonus: after just five months of shielding my right (dominant) arm from danger I am becoming ambidextrous. I can now iron, polish shoes, brush my teeth, butter bread and take a roast from the oven with the wrong arm. Something else to put on my CV.

J is for journey

You are not going into hospital – you are going on a journey. Hospital folk love the term *the Patient Journey*. I think we are supposed to believe that we are not alone, that the process is being *mapped* (see what they're doing there –

maps, journeys – see?). Journey suggests to me a clear route, a flowing, continuous pathway, an excursion. It sounds almost pleasant. And I've heard they have other daft terms too, like *care delivery system* and *patient journey management system*. I liked it better when we were just plain old doctor and patient. And what's next? Will the doctors become service providers, treatment facilitators, journey navigators? The Patient Journey; spare me. Across the Styx, maybe. Well, let me tell you about my journey: no one seems to be driving the bus and no matter how much I ring the bell, I can't get off.

I say all this not just because I find the term 'the Patient Journey' more than a teensy bit patronising, but because even though I know the NHS genuinely strives to make 'continuity of care' more than just an alliterative illusion, you may find yourself stumbling, punch drunk, from one department to the next. And while each one may do a really excellent job, you can't help wondering, Who's in charge?

In some health trusts the doublespeak is taken a step further. You are not a patient, you are a *client*. Seriously, I hate that – I am not waiting in the foyer of an advertising agency. I am not going to have my nails done. 'Client' supposedly destigmatises us and makes it seem like we have more say in what is happening to us than we really do – like we are entering into a business deal and we could just get up and take our 'custom' elsewhere. Perhaps language has evolved too far.

Maybe we need to take a step backwards: you doctor; me sick. You make sick better. Yes?

Top tip: don't pay the ferryman until he gets you to the other side.

J is for jokes

Until I only had one, I never noticed just how many jokes, verbal and visual, make reference to breasts. From *Carry On* movies to TV sitcoms, the breast is an object of good-natured fun. When you are fresh from your mastectomy this can make you feel a bit left out. Don't these people realise we don't all have a matching set?

And then there are all the bad-taste jokes about cancer. I saw two of these in the weeks following my operation (serves me right for watching E4) and I came over all indignant and self-righteous. Then, a few weeks later, I found myself watching the politically incorrect satirical comedy *Thank You for Smoking* about the tobacco industry trying to prove that smoking and lung cancer are unrelated. It is shameless but hilarious. I also found myself roaring with laughter at a *Mitchell and Webb* sketch where one man tells another of his cancer at his wedding. Hysterical. Thank you TV for reminding me that I have a sense of humour.

So remember, they have removed your boob, not your personality. Let yourself laugh.

K is for knickers

You need your sense of humour for this one.

For the final weeks of my radiotherapy and for two months afterwards, I wore knickers where I should have worn a bra. My skin was at first too damaged, and then too easily bruised to wear even the recommended nuns' bras. I had dressings over the entire breast area and up into the armpit, and these dressings needed to be held in place by some non-adhesive method. 'Have you tried our bras?' the radiotherapy nurse said, brandishing one such garment before me.

'Aren't they old people's knickers used to keep incontinence pads in place?' I asked.

She didn't admit it, but you could see from her face that she'd been found out. She took the soft, mesh knickers, cut a V in the crotch, turned them upside down and hey presto – a bra-type garment that is not only comfortable but keeps your dressings in position too. Your head comes out the crotch and your arms come out the leg holes. Ingenious.

K is for keeping it real

If you are not careful, you could end up living in a parallel universe where the only thing that exists is cancer, so you will have to make an enormous effort to keep things real.

Following a week-long stay in hospital, I was discharged at 2.30 p.m. and I wanted to go straight home to bed and lick my wounds. But school let out at 3 p.m., so instead of going for my lie-down I went and collected my son from school. You should have seen his face light up when he saw me. I was back in the real world.

It is an effort to keep doing things, especially when you are exhausted. And then there is the added problem of feeling a bit feeble-minded at this time. A few times when people asked me to do things I would think, I can't do that – I have cancer; or I can't do that – I only have one boob. When really, there was no good reason why I couldn't help out – I just felt out of kilter with the world. Well, the only way to get back in kilter is to do things. And so I put a toe back into the world and found myself selling raffle tickets for the music school, driving the ten-year-old and his mates to a swimming gala and taking part in a 'Ceremony of Light' when my radio-therapy burns were so bad that the nurse told me not to. I only did it because my son pleaded with me. He was sick of having a sick mum. So I did it. I stood at the front of the church and lit the candles the children brought to me and felt choked when I had to light the candle of one child whose mother had died of breast cancer a few years before. That was hard.

These things may not seem much, but they were such a big deal to me at the time. However, they were worth it. It is really important to come down from planet cancer and do these ordinary everyday things, even if it feels impossible. For me, one of the biggest hurdles was dressing up for Halloween as it came only weeks after my mastectomy. We dress up every year, but this time I told everyone I wouldn't be partying and in fact, no one expected me to. Then, as I was smearing green face paint and fake blood on my son's face I thought, *If I don't go to this party, cancer really is spoiling my life, and his.* That was it; I was going, but I only had fifteen minutes to get ready. With my post-operative paleness and a daft wig, I went as a (not very convincing) Amy Winehouse, wearing a black mini dress, black tights and black knee-high boots. At the party one of the other mums asked me if I'd hired my costume from the fancy-dress shop downtown. 'No,' I told her. 'These are my clothes.'

Maybe I need to keep the wardrobe real too.

L is for lymphoedema

If you are having your lymph nodes removed (see ANC, page 10) or radiotherapy to your armpit you will be told about the risk of lymphoedema. Or at least you should be. Oedema simply means swelling – in this case due to an excess of lymph fluid in your arm. I am told that the fluid builds up because the lymph nodes have been removed or have become blocked due to radiotherapy and the drainage system can't work properly any more. The breast care nurse made this amply clear to me right from the start and I remember thinking, So my arm will swell up. So? I'll be alive, right? Faced with a choice between cancer and a fat arm, you'd choose the fat arm any day. However, the risk of lymphoedema is lifelong, so you should take seriously the advice they give you on trying to reduce yours.

The lymphatic system helps fight infection, so the best thing to do is to put as little strain on the system as possible. That is why they give you such thorough advice on avoiding infection (see page 114). They also recommend exercises and keeping the area well moisturised. If you do get lymphoedema they will provide you with a compression garment (a bit like the dreaded flight socks – see page 99) to wear over the arm, and they may offer you manual lymphatic drainage – a highly specialised massage technique that helps drain fluid.

When I first mentioned that I was concerned that I might

be getting lymphoedema a nurse said to me, 'There is a society for that, you know.' And I said, 'What, like the choral society?' We had a bit of a laugh over that, but really, I didn't want support – I wanted to be checked out. Frustrated, I went back to the physio who was dealing with my cording. She took out a tape measure and noted that yes, there was a slight difference in the girth of my arms and referred me on to the correct department. I was then seen very promptly, so they evidently take the problem seriously. So should you.

L is for looking good

This is not the time to start neglecting yourself. Cancer treatments take their toll and I found I had to work extra hard just to look OK. I know some people will say, so what – if you can't look rough now, when can you? But I disagree, and I am not just being vain and frivolous here.

My looking good was important for my son too. So just forty minutes after being brought back from surgery I was applying make-up with a very shaky hand to mask the dark circles under my eyes and to dot some colour on my pale, post-operative cheeks and lips. And all this so that the ten-year-old would not be frightened witless at the sight of me. Remember, I had a drip, three drains and one of those nasal canula tube things. I'd also turned down a pre-med before the operation because I didn't want to be too 'out of it' when he came to see me. And it all worked: his first words when he came in that evening were, 'You don't look too bad, actually.'

People will say you have better things to think about at a time like this, but remember, looking good makes you *feel* good; it makes you feel able to face the world. And it's not just a matter of make-up. You might never have worn make-up in your life, and you don't have to start now, but there are other steps you can take to look good.

When I was a student in the eighties I was heavily influenced by women who made me feel intellectually and morally inferior for wearing make-up. I was seen as frivolous, an intellectual lightweight (apparently lipstick interferes with brain functioning). Well, now that I am old and ugly enough to know better, I am not going to let latter-day worthies make me feel bad about trying to feel good.

One of the last things I did before I went in for my mastectomy was to dye my hair, even though it was presumed at that point that I'd be having chemotherapy and was therefore about to lose it all. I reckoned I only had about a month or so left with my hair and I wanted it to look normal; once you start letting the roots show, the nails chip and the belly sag you are going down a sorry route at the end of which bad breath and depression await. You will look bad and feel bad and a nasty little voice in your head will tell you that the cancer is getting the better of you. Don't let it.

And so I want to applaud the cosmetics industry – and although, no doubt, some smarty pants could write a paper on how it preys on the vulnerabilities of cancer patients, locking them into a cycle of dependency and demand for their products, I say pish* to that. The cosmetics industry runs a scheme for women with cancer called 'Look Good ... Feel Better', whereby they are invited to attend a beauty session at which they are given free advice on skincare and (for those experiencing hair loss) tips on tying bandanas and drawing in missing eyebrows. Looking and feeling good is especially challenging for women going through chemo and, I think, especially important. So much of what you see as your femininity has been stripped away, those things that help define you: your breasts, your lovely eyelashes, that head of hair ... So a treat like this is really valuable.

When I went for my session, only one woman there was in a bandana and after the session she was the most transformed. And not because she had a pile of slap on, but because she was being made to *feel* beautiful. (God, I'm beginning to sound like a commercial.) And it doesn't end there. They give you a seriously luscious goody bag (full of

---

*This is an exclamation of contempt used since the 1500s and beloved of Shakespeare and has nothing to do with urinating. I checked.

things I couldn't afford) and qualified beauticians show you how to use it all properly. You get a cup of tea too, have a laugh and it is all free. It definitely made me feel good.

I found out about it through my local cancer charity and was disappointed at first that there was such a long waiting list. But don't be put off. Long after treatment has ended you will still need a boost.

L is for lone parent

Let's get one thing straight. Not all lone parents are the benefit-scrounging, beer-drinking, chip-eating slobs the media would have you believe. Some of us don't even watch daytime TV. Some of us are quite nice, actually.

Getting a diagnosis of cancer was the only time I really worried about being a lone parent. Before that, I smugly looked on as some two-parent units fought over how best to discipline little Tarquin. They always seemed to be contradicting each other and confusing the child – bickering about how best to bring him up, blaming each other for mistakes. Blame doesn't exist in the same way for a lone parent. Responsibility does. And getting cancer only highlights that, to the extent that for once I thought I'd been irresponsible in bringing up this child on my own. But then I wised up. You cannot stay with someone just in case you get sick some time down the line. Then I thought, maybe I was irresponsible for not trying harder to find a new mate and replacement dad. Too late now though. What would I put on my internet profile? Single white female, good sense of humour, one boob . . .

Look for the small mercies: at least you don't have to worry about your husband worrying. And let's face it, that's probably what would happen. You know you'd end up looking after him, making sure he didn't get too stressed, trying not to wake him when you cry at night, keeping his spirits up. Poor love.

As a lone parent you can devote all your attention to keeping your own and the children's spirits up. Far better.

PS OK, yes, I do consume chips and beer sometimes.

L is for lottery

After years of stubbornly refusing to play the lottery I have joined the poor deluded masses who sit home on a Saturday night waiting, dreaming. I didn't do it before on the grounds that the government already gets loads of my cash in the form of taxes. Why would I want to give them any more in a daft draw that I had next to no hope of winning? Besides,

I reckoned the more money we gave the lottery, the more the government had to spend on weapons and warmongering, and I didn't want that on my conscience. But now that my future seems precarious (I am on half pay and don't know when I'll get back to work) my conscience has shrunk and I feel the need to become an instant millionaire.

When I first heard Jade Goody's justification for televising her cancer – that she only wanted to pay for her boys' education – I was sniffy. Hadn't she heard that primary and secondary education are free in the UK? And even if the boys decided to go on to third-level education, it wouldn't take several millions to cover the cost. Now, however, I think about my own son's future and I think, Yup, he will need loads of money and I may not be able to work to provide it ...

So ... it's Saturday today. Lotto day. You never know ...

M is for mastectomy

I'd never had an ectomy before. They were always something that happened to other people, and on TV. I thought of my school days when tonsillectomies were all the rage and remembered how envious I was of my friends eating ice cream in a hospital bed away from teachers and homework. It never occurred to me to consider why they were having the operation in the first place or worry that those tonsils might actually have had a use.

Now I am grown up I don't see hospital as an ice-cream-filled holiday. I knew *this* ectomy meant cancer and was fairly sure I could use both my breasts, thanks. Yet when the surgeon said she was planning to do a total mastectomy I didn't complain. I was relieved. In theory, it would have been comforting to hear that I only needed a partial mastectomy or lumpectomy because then I could tell myself things weren't so bad, and I'd still have two boobs. But you've probably noted by now that I am a little inclined to worry and I just know that had she performed a partial mastectomy I'd be going around worrying: did she miss a bit?

You'll be glad to hear that they take your cancer and some more; that's what they mean when they talk about clear margins. Sometimes this might not be possible. In my case, not all the margins were satisfactory because one lump was so close to my chest wall. As one nurse put it, if they'd taken any more my lungs would've fallen out. Some might think that a bit glib, but I liked its honest simplicity. I understood. And I'm quite sure she had me sussed and knew a joke wouldn't go amiss. Horses for courses.

Once you've been told you are going to have a mastectomy, things move quickly so you don't have much time to think. I was so preoccupied with the notion of getting this cancer cut out that it never occurred to me to fully consider what I would actually look like after the operation. The nurse had shown me photographs of women who'd had reconstructive surgery, but I never really identified with them. Somehow, I would look better than them, with maybe a flat, nipple-free area and a neat line of stitches. I didn't expect a big scar because the only operation I'd had before was a Caesarean and the scar is minute. I thought that if they can get an eight-and-a-half-pound baby out and leave barely a trace, then surely a boob wouldn't cause too much mess. I was wrong.

You might be anxious about looking at yourself after the operation. I know many women are, but I was curious to see my surgeon's handiwork. The day after the operation I took myself off to the shower room and peeled back the dressing to see a large, and what I can only describe as bumpy, scar. There appeared to be leftover bits of nipple knotted into what seemed to me a very long and twisted line of stitches. Hadn't the surgeon told me there was a lump just behind the nipple? Had she forgotten? Oh my God! She had missed a bit.

I stayed in the shower room hyperventilating for a while, then went back to my bed for a lie-down and a cry. I'd only been there a few minutes when (thank you God) one of the registrars came along on his rounds. He bent over me and peered at the scar, 'Looks like a skin-saving technique,' he said. And he was right. The surgeon hadn't missed anything: I'd had a 'skin-sparing' mastectomy, which meant that most of my skin was retained (complete with tan lines from the summer). She had also removed the nipple, but left the areola. How clever is that? I imagined the surgeon slicing open the skin, scooping out the offending tissue like the filling of a jacket potato gone rotten and stitching me up again. I wondered if she was any good in the kitchen.

About a week after the operation my skin bloomed with purple and yellow bruises that I had not expected. These bruises upset me. I felt shocked and upset and really stupid. How had I not expected bruising? The bruises took a few weeks to disappear, but the scar took longer. It went through a strange process – an unfurling. What I had thought of as chewed-up bits of nipple revealed themselves to be a healthy-looking areola, a bit squished, but quite nice, actually. Meanwhile, the line of stitches disappeared almost completely, leaving the shortest crease, barely visible. Honest to God, the craftsmanship is so impressive that I feel like showing it off. Almost.

I almost went for mastectomy without reconstruction because it is so much simpler. It means less time under anaesthetic, shorter recovery time and fewer potential complications. It also means no implants (which, incidentally, are only expected to last about fifteen years). I know some women who opted for mastectomy only and I can understand that. They are happy with their decision and with the prosthesis (fake boob) they have been given. I was initially attracted to the mastectomy-only route because at that moment in time I wasn't thinking, Oh poor me and my boob – I was thinking, Get this thing off me. In the end, however, I opted for a tissue expander (see page 177).

This is the area of treatment where you have possibly the most say and the breast care nurses are brilliant with their advice and information. But the decision is yours. Go with your instinct; it will tell you what to do.

M is for men

Men get breast cancer too; around 400 men are diagnosed with it in the UK every year. Now that really is cruel. It means that not only do they have to come to terms with cancer, but also with the fact that they have breasts they never knew they had. It must be so hard for a man to say the words 'I have breast cancer'. You can just hear the locker-room jibes and the bad-taste jokes. I think that doctors should spare these men their blushes and invent a new term for male breast cancer. (Best not to leave it to the people who named the Cancer Centre though – see E is for euphemisms.)

There is also a link between breast cancer in men and prostate cancer. I suppose it's all hormone related. Anyway, if you know someone with a prostate problem, make sure they take seriously any changes in their nipples – male breast cancer is often found just around the nipple.

N is for nurses

A childhood friend of mine went on to become a nurse and seeing the work she did gave me a lifelong respect for the profession. I really don't know how they do it, and no, I don't think they get paid enough.

I received excellent nursing care, both in hospital and as an outpatient. The nurses were kind and funny (even when giving an enema). If I have any criticism to make it is only that they are so busy attending to process – making sure that early-warning charts are filled in, regulations met, drugs doled out on schedule – that they may miss the chance to care for the *person*. Don't get me wrong, those practical tasks are crucially important, but my concern is that, over time, old-fashioned 'And-how-are-you-today-dear?' nursing will disappear.

There must be bad nurses, just like there are bad teachers, plumbers, politicians, but thankfully, I never met any of them. Yes, I was annoyed by that first nurse who couldn't hide her irritation and kept on telling me I was 'taking this badly' (see page 13). But even though she annoyed me, she still did a really good job. And anyway, I refuse to let that one experience colour my judgement of everyone else.

I am sure my surgery was made bearable because the nurses prepared me so well. And I know that the ordeal of radiotherapy would have been intolerable were it not for the ministrations and sense of fun of the radiotherapy nurses. You'd think that working with cancer every day would leave nurses numbed to its full horrors, like teenage boys playing Grand Theft Auto who are desensitised to violence, but that doesn't seem to be the case. Somehow, in spite of seeing sickness every day, good nurses still manage to care about you and make you feel like you matter.

One nurse especially stands out. She was the perfect combination of efficiency and compassion. And she was firm too. After a mastectomy there is a tendency to overprotect your bad arm. You naturally shield it and hold it in an injured pose. This is bad: you have to get it moving naturally or more problems can set in. I remember this particular nurse being very firm with me about this, but in a helpful way. She was just really good at her job. She managed to combine all the chart-ticking, drug-doling, obs-taking, drip-checking stuff with listening and really engaging with the patients. She was the one who told me it was important to cry, and she was also the one I turned to when fear threatened to choke me. When, on the night of my operation, I told her I was afraid to go to sleep because my sister had suffered brain-stem injury the night they operated on her tumour, she knew, as I did, that I was being irrational. She knew that I wasn't going to die in the night. She knew that I was visiting a place from the past full of fear and sadness and despair, and so she rested her hand on my arm and said she'd look after me. And she did. She came regularly through the night doing obs and asking how I was. I barely slept and her presence comforted me. And that is what nursing is all about.

N is for nursing pads

Nursing pads are soft disposable discs made to slip inside the bras of breastfeeding mothers to soak up any milk that leaks out between feeds. I wore these while breastfeeding, otherwise I'd have looked like a competitor in a wet T-shirt competition. Not a good look when you're pushing a trolley round Sainsbury's. Due to my cancer treatment, I felt too uncomfortable to wear bras and so wore soft tops and vests. These were practical, but not very flattering, especially as the one remaining nipple stood to attention through the too-soft material, drawing the eye to it and thence to the other impoverished boob.

Lay folk don't tend to discriminate between their nipple and their areola (the dark bumpy skin surrounding the nipple); it's all one and the same to most of us. However, with certain surgical procedures it is possible to have the nipple removed and the areola saved. I had this and now that the wound is healed and the scar shrunk to near invisible, I am impressed with the result. However, my 'nipples' are not symmetrical; one looks like a raspberry, all ripe and ready, and the other looks like a raspberry that some rotter has trodden on. Until such time as I can wear a padded bra, the difference is visible through T-shirts and jumpers. Thank goodness, then, for nursing pads. I can slip these in under my top to produce a smoother, more symmetrical outline. Don't know why no one thought of it before.

N is for nipple

If you don't fancy nipple reconstruction (see B is for breast reconstruction, page 25) and nursing pads feel too mumsy for you, you could opt for stick-on nipples. The breast care nurse told me about these on my second visit to the clinic. Stick-on nipples. I couldn't concentrate. Sure, you might look good in a T-shirt, but what happens when you want to 'get jiggy with it'. Would the nipples stay on or would the phrase, 'Do you swallow?' take on a whole new meaning?

O is for other cancers

Do not freak out every time your doctor has you tested for another cancer. A good doctor should be a professional hypochondriac; it is their job to worry and fuss over your health. They would be negligent, given your history, if they didn't check out any suspicious symptoms you develop.

Luckily, my GP told me right at the start that for years to come every twinge would be investigated with cancer in mind, so I wasn't shocked or horrified when I was sent home with a hideous little kit used to screen for bowel cancer. (The kit detects *Fecal Occult Blood*. Sounds like a video nasty, some kitsch 1970s' devil-worship horror. And no, it is nothing like a home pregnancy-testing kit; for a start, you have to bring it back to the lab for analysis – ick, who'd work in a lab? – and then there is the agonising wait for your results.)

If they found your nodes were affected by the primary cancer, you will have been given extra tests and scans to determine whether or not the cancer has spread to other areas of the body. This can provide peace of mind if you get the 'all clear', and the reassurance that something will be done if you do not. Look on testing for other cancers as an opportunity, not a threat. And if fear makes you falter, remember the mantra: early diagnosis saves lives.

P is for positive mental attitude

'I am a great believer in PMA,' the breast care nurse said to me as I sat before her bawling my eyes out. PMA? I had no idea what she meant. I thought maybe it was some kind of drug treatment. (Cancer is full of acronyms and abbreviations: CAT scan, TRAM flap, ANC, HER2 – the list goes on.) I considered the possible meanings. Hmm, I wondered ... PMA – post-mammogram angst (I've got that in spades)? Pre-menopausally acquired? Poly-mastic appendage? All wrong. The reality was much simpler: it is positive mental attitude, as if you could just *think* the cancer away!

They talk about PMA a lot, as if cancer was a scourge sent to teach all the miserable old pessimists a lesson. PMA! I really had no idea what that meant, and I almost wish I hadn't asked, because now I have to pretend to be cheerful all the time or the cancer will somehow be my own fault. Something else to feel guilty about.

See also T is for trust.

P is for privacy

Forget it: you won't get any in an NHS hospital. I was admitted to a mixed ward the night before my operation and then transferred to the correct ward the following morning. This presumably had to do with the pressure on beds. I didn't particularly like it, but I didn't mind it either; I was just grateful they were seeing me so promptly. My blind panic had been replaced by a calm that was far more irrational than any other emotion I'd experienced so far. I was in hospital and they were going to fix me. I lay there with the bed curtains drawn round me listening to snippets of information about the other people on the ward. It was better than an episode of *Holby*. Mrs X's medication needed to be changed. Mr Y was back: his ninety-seventh overdose that year. Ninety-seven! Someone made a sick joke about practice making perfect, and I wondered if anyone had made some bad-taste joke about me. I heard that one person was ready for discharge, another for transfer, that the Breast Lady needed her bloods done. Wait a minute. The Breast Lady. That was me.

Try really hard to steel yourself against the loss of privacy that being in an NHS hospital entails. You can draw the curtains around you, but you cannot keep the news within them. Newsflash: sound travels through fabric.

P is for perspiration

You've heard of eating for two, well my 'good' armpit is sweating for two. The armpit that was operated on doesn't sweat at all now, but the other one more than makes up for it. I am not used to this. I have never been a Sweaty Betty, but now I have expansive unilateral sweat stains. Honestly, if you were a symmetry freak, you just couldn't cope. I blame the Tamoxifen for my increased sweating as I stubbornly refuse to believe it is just me.

Meanwhile, the radiation seems to have had a permanent depilatory effect on the 'bad' armpit. Imagine – hair removal as a cosmetic spin-off from radiotherapy. Sound scary? (The ten-year-old tells me that when radium was discovered it was used to brighten complexions and make teeth glow, but only until they realised it could kill you.)

P is for prosthesis

I find the word prosthesis difficult. It makes me think of detachable limbs and 'creeps me out', as the ten-year-old would say.

A breast prosthesis is an artificial boob that fits inside your bra and replaces the missing one. It makes me think of those schoolgirls who shoved tissues down their bras to make themselves seem better endowed. It feels fake. That is one of the benefits of going for reconstructive surgery; you bypass all of this conflict. Lucky me. But when my reconstructive surgery was postponed and I had to get back to work – well, I couldn't go with just one boob, could I? So they fitted me with a prosthesis. And you know what? It's not half bad.

Unfortunately, the same could not be said of the temporary 'prosthesis' I was given just before I left hospital. It was what they call a *softie*, and I can honestly say it was about as effective as a rolled-up sock. Not only that, it was edged with blanket stitch (in what appeared to be nylon thread) and my skin was so sensitive that every single stitch left an indentation. The boob looked like pastry that had been crimped with a fork, ready for the oven. Worse still, these 'softies' are OK so long as you don't actually move, at which point they pop out and it's red faces all round. I tried wearing mine half a dozen times or so, then I just gave up and covered up.

When I was finally able to wear a bra, the breast care nurse fitted me with a non-wired, wide-strapped, deep-sided, full-cupped monstrosity that you'd expect your granny to wear – and it felt just perfect. I knew I needed one of these, I just hadn't known where to get my hands on one. All the bra shops I'd formerly frequented only seemed to offer skimpy, underwired, skinny-strapped bras, so I was delighted with the nurse's range of 'old lady' bras. Once the bra was sorted, the nurse produced the prosthesis. A squishy, silicone (I think) moulded form that fits inside the pocket of the bra. I believe these types of breast forms are similar to the chicken fillets some regular, double-breasted women wear to give themselves *an advantage*. I've always thought the idea of stuffing chicken fillets down your bra so you can look like Pamela Anderson absurd and a bit of a cheat. What happens when you get the man those boobs have won you home? How does he cope with the disappointment? (Imagine if men stuffed chicken fillets down their Y-fronts . . .)

The breast care nurse also gave me a catalogue featuring glamorous mastectomy bras for *that special occasion*. I told her I wasn't ever planning on having special occasions again, not ever. Never. And she said to me, 'Do not close the door on opportunity.' I didn't tell her (in case she berated me for my lack of PMA), but I had the feeling that opportunity had just closed the door on me.

Now that I am single breasted, however, I feel justified in using 'fakes' and I don't see it as artifice; I see it as an anatomical necessity. These fake boobs are brilliant. Or at least mine is. The bra and the prosthesis felt odd and a bit uncomfortable to begin with and the nurse advised me to 'build up' wear, a bit like getting used to contact lenses, I suppose. This wasn't really necessary in my case as I soon adjusted to the feel and the weight of it, but I suppose it's a different story for large-breasted women. For them, the weight of the fake boob could be substantial, and since it isn't actually attached to your body, it could pull down and away when you bend over. Does this have implications for lymphoedema sufferers? God, there is so much to worry about ... But apart from that, my final verdict on breast prostheses is that while they are not perfect, they are really very good indeed. I can see why people just go with them and forget about further surgery.

NB Some charities offer excellent bra-fitting services, but my advice is to wait until well after surgery – especially recon-structive surgery – as these bras are expensive and you want to get it right. I also found you can buy less expensive versions of post-surgery bras from some stores.

P is for probably

I know that there are both art and science (and maybe even a bit of educated guesswork) in good doctoring, but if I hear one more doctor say, 'That's probably the radiotherapy', I'll scream.

Radiotherapy is the bogeyman that gets blamed for every ache, swelling, itching, reddening or bit of discomfort that you experience for months and (I'm told) years after therapy has ended. My collarbone had a swelling on one side. It was accompanied by a bruised feeling and though slight, it was obvious enough for the ten-year-old to notice. 'It's probably the radiotherapy' two doctors told me, one after the other. 'What *probably* is the radiotherapy doing to my collarbone?' I wanted to scream. Had it altered my DNA for good? Was I becoming a mutant? I was fairly sure I wouldn't end up like Quasimodo, but *probably* just wasn't enough, not where cancer was concerned. I needed something a bit more definitive.

I braced myself and asked politely if the doctor could find out for sure what the problem was, all the while thinking (and I am not proud of this), You don't have to go to medical school to tell me what it 'probably' is; the ten-year-old could do that. But I kept the thought to myself. There was nothing to be gained by being rude. Learn from me; my restraint worked: the doctor ordered an X-ray. And it came back normal.

Probably just the radiotherapy, then.

P is for pyjamas

A friend told me a story of when her mother-in-law used to come and stay from time to time, and how, one night, they bumped into each other as they both stumbled, bleary-eyed, to the bathroom. Through the mother-in-law's soft, flowing nightie my friend noticed that she had only one breast, and was shocked, as her husband had never mentioned it. So she did some digging. It transpired that her mother-in-law had had a mastectomy when her boys were young and had decided not to tell them. She still hadn't said a word even though the 'boys' were now both nearing forty. Needless to say, after that night, the skeleton was out of the cupboard.

The moral of this story is, if you don't want people to notice your mastectomy, don't wear soft, flowing nighties. The eye is drawn to the imbalance. When I was admitted to hospital for my mastectomy I was upset by the sight of the woman in the bed opposite; the soft folds of her very nice nightie clung to her one remaining boob, screaming out that the other one was missing.

Thank goodness I had already bought cotton pyjamas with button-through jackets which were much more discreet. The material doesn't cling, you see. They don't have to be armour, just good-quality cotton. And you don't have to spend a fortune. You can buy PJs in most large supermarkets nowadays, but make sure you don't buy anything too flimsy, as they might be a bit transparent. Button-through pyjama jackets have the added bonus of sparing your blushes when the doctor comes round. You can quickly unbutton the jacket and slip one shoulder down, whereas with a nightie you have to pull the whole blinkin' thing up from your knees. Not dignified.

P is for poetry

You might find yourself coming over all poetic at a time like this.

A few days after my diagnosis I remember sitting in the car, watching the late September sunlight dapple the leaves of a chestnut tree ... Enough.

Seriously though, cancer brings life into sharp focus, and you might find yourself noticing and relishing every little detail, then feeling the need to write about it. And judging from the number of people signing up for creative writing classes at my local cancer charity, creative expression is very important and useful at a time like this. So go on, explore your creative side. Because poetry is good for your soul. It stirs and it soothes. I gave up praying in favour of poetry a very long time ago, and when I need comfort that's what I turn to. Right now, I find myself coming back to that famous Dylan Thomas villanelle about his father dying: 'Do Not Go Gentle Into That Good Night'. I keep saying it over and over, like a prayer.

Do not go gentle into that good night ...

Q is for queer-sounding words

The other day the ten-year-old smirked at me over his favourite science book and said, 'Do you know what a contusion to the gluteus maximus is?'

Well, do you?

There is nothing wrong with stopping your doctor to say that you do not understand what he is talking about. Just be straight. Say, 'What do you mean?' plain and simple. Of course, you could say, 'What *exactly* do you mean?' if your vanity is such that you want to appear as though you only partially don't understand. I don't recommend this, however, because it suggests a certain level of comprehension on your part and you cannot blame the doctor if he doesn't realise *exactly* which bit you don't get. Keep it simple and ask when you don't know, otherwise a bruise on the bum could get awfully complicated.

Q is for questions

Remember how I said that cancer had an infantilising effect on me, making me huff like a toddler, squawking, 'No!' at my surgeon? Well, it wasn't long before my infantilised self added a new word to my vocabulary – *Why?*

I remembered back to when the ten-year-old was a toddler pestering me with *whys*. Why is rain wet? Why do dogs bark? Why can't we poke a hole in gravity, so we can all float about? (Seriously, he did ask me that.) Now I am that toddler, asking 'Why?' all the time. Why, why, why? But why? I am confounded and tormented by my own ignorance. Just as well then, that before you meet your doctors, the nurses will urge you to write down all your questions in readiness. They might even give you some information booklets which have special sections at the back, with blank lines for your Q&As. And if you are completely clueless like me, this is a brilliant idea.

So on the night before my first oncology appointment I jotted down nearly twenty questions. And these were only the ones I knew to ask. I had loads more; I just didn't know what they were yet. When you don't know your axilla from your anus, it's hard to formulate a meaningful question. Still, the doctor would explain and then I'd know.

That first oncology appointment was a big deal. I was terrified, but I was also relieved, having been led to believe that the oncologist would take control, listen to my questions and answer them all. And so I approached my oncology appointment like King Arthur's knights approaching the Holy Grail. All would be revealed, right? I took out my piece of paper and a pen to write down the answers and started my quest. What causes cancer? Are there any alternatives to Tamoxifen?

Will my tissue expander affect my radiotherapy treatment? Do hospital budgets affect the treatment I get? Could pre-cancerous cells on my chest wall mutate and migrate to my lungs and set up a colony there? And what *is* cancer, anyway? But the registrar seemed uneasy discussing these things with me, and the consultant seemed under pressure of time, so I ended up feeling like a nuisance with my questions.

And I was embarrassed too (other patients told me they felt equally awkward). When I took out my pen and paper I felt like a hypochondriac with a fetish for dictation and I was terrified that the doctor was thinking, Oh God, here we go. We've got a right one here. I imagined him scribbling little coded acronyms and abbreviations at the top of my notes for future reference: ANT (annoying note-taker), PIN (pain in neck).

It struck me that I hadn't felt like this during my surgical consultation, and that doctor seemed to be under just as much pressure, with an equally full waiting room. So what was the difference? The only obvious difference that I can spot (apart from the personalities involved) is the breast care nurses. At my surgical consultation, the breast care nurse stepped in and filled in all the blanks, explained all the tricky bits, then let me have a good cry. These nurses do such a good job that you are bereft without them. At least, I was.

The problem is that, even if they wanted to, doctors simply don't have the time to anticipate and respond to all our questions. Try and put yourself in their shoes. These people are under pressure and waiting lists are long. Doctors have heavy workloads and busy schedules. I understand that they have unrealistic targets that have been set by managers who, I believe, know precious little about doctoring. We cannot presume that doctors will readily invite questions. But we must still keep asking.

So however awkward it may make you feel, the best way round the problem is to prepare for each appointment as though it were a world summit. Have your aims and objectives, your desired outcomes, all thought out. Write them all down if you have to and be resolute. And don't be shy about producing your notes at a consultation. It'll be an exhausting – almost Sisyphean – task, but it should help you optimise your time with the doctor. Maybe you are good at getting to the nub of things in a brief hospital appointment, but I'm not. I need written notes because either my mind empties or it fills up with junk, and I suffer from a kind of delayed reaction, whereby I process what they are saying five minutes after they've said it and it's too late. Like the time I went to the doctor with breast pain (in the remaining boob) and he told me he wouldn't organise a mammogram because nothing would happen in the year between my scheduled scans. I was dressed and he had gone before I had the chance to say, 'Well heck, that's just not true ...' Unless we are to believe that just having a mammogram provides a twelve-month prophylactic effect, the lump has to start growing at some point in the calendar year. You'll hear of lots of people who developed tumours in between scans. I myself had an 'all-clear' scan ten months prior to the mammogram that detected my malignant lump. So I think what the doctor really meant was that it was not procedure or even wise to offer impromptu scans. That seems reasonable to me, but if that is the case, just say it.

I blame myself. I took my eye off the ball. (Which is why just preparing in advance is not enough – you have to stay focused, and that way you know that you haven't wasted their time or your own. And when this works, it is brilliant.) Feeling confused and unsatisfied after that meeting, I promptly spoke to another doctor in the clinic who went out of her way to set my mind at ease. She didn't give me a scan – she explained why I wasn't getting one and what might be the cause of my pain. She was brilliant. But it wouldn't have happened if I hadn't asked. So, the moral of the story is . . . *ASK*!

You may have to be really persistent with your questions, and some doctors may not always thank you for your curiosity. But the consultant dermatologist I went to see about my radiotherapy burns told me never to stop asking questions. And while this may mean becoming unpopular with some people, here's the thing: cancer is not a popularity contest. Cancer is a matter of life and death. KOA. Keep on asking.

R is for relationships

This is where the clichés really take hold – 'You find out who your friends are', 'You see people in their true colours', 'Blood is thicker than water' (but only sometimes).

Following a cancer diagnosis the world will for ever after be split into two camps: those who supported you through the experience, and those who did not. The trick here is to stay focused on the supporters: those who rushed in with practical, emotional and even financial support; those who wore their knees out praying for you or put up with your moods and your misery.

But you should also know this: cancer does not turn mean people nice. On the day I was diagnosed I thought, Oh God, here we go, everyone is going to go all earnest on me and start being nice all the time. Ha! I couldn't have been more wrong. If you have a colleague or friend or relation who is cold and unfeeling, you having cancer will not make them less so. If you have a boss who is a mean-minded bully, you having cancer won't change that. I also naively thought cancer could bring families together, make them all chummy, you know, like *The Waltons*. But I've since heard so many stories of family fall-outs that I now know better. I have even heard of people crossing the street to avoid speaking to someone with cancer. And none of the leaflets prepare you for that.

It needs to be said that a cancer diagnosis can cause seismic shifts to occur in your relationships, and the sad thing is that the gaps left behind may never be filled. When you have cancer you see your relationships with a new clarity. I see such warmth and generosity in some, such goodness; but I also see the other side. I see the absentees and the wrongdoers. Those people who stayed away and stayed silent. Or worse, used my weakened state to settle an ancient grudge.

Luckily, most of those around me showed their 'true colours' to be good, kind and generous. And yet I am left with the bitterness of those who did not. And it hurts. I think people need to know that when you have cancer, you feel that hurt more acutely. So while it's true to say that I remember every kindness that people did for me – the soups made, the time spent, the hands held – I can't help but also remember every single wound too.

And I see myself more clearly too. I see that I may sometimes have hurt people by pushing away their attempts to help me, not because I was too proud or was being *brave*, but simply because I'm used to doing things for myself, and letting these helpers in was like letting the cancer in too – acknowledging the gravity of the situation.

So yes, some of your relationships will suffer from your diagnosis of cancer. Some people will try, but fail to deal with it. Some will deny or diminish your experience. And some will manage, through an impressive feat of egotism, to make *your* cancer about *them*. (I don't know why they do this. I bet psychologists have a field day concocting theories about this, and why some people shun and punish you for having cancer. But you know what? I don't want to understand.)

You have to learn the art of self-preservation. And hopefully, for every one person that hurts you, there will be two that help. Don't lose sight of that. Better still, some of your relationships will be even stronger than before and that can only be a good thing. And best of all, cancer didn't make these people nice. They were nice before.

R is for reflex action

I consider myself a reasonably reasonable sort of person. I admit to occasionally lashing out with second-rate sarcasm, but I don't usually swear at people and I certainly don't hit people, especially those who are trying to help me. So my urge to slap the face of the young nurse who removed my final chest drain after the mastectomy was shocking.

I am still appalled by the force of the feeling. I was a bit nervous about getting the third and final drain out. Like a wimp, I'd asked for, but had been refused painkillers. (Still don't see the sense in that.) The first drain came out shortly after the operation, while I was still receiving intravenous pain relief, so I didn't feel much. The second was uncomfortable, but nothing to write home about. But the third! Maybe if the nurse had warned me; maybe if she'd given me the painkillers I'd asked for . . .

Now, I know that the nurse (who was very nice, incidentally) was only doing her job, but the experience was such an affront that I just wanted to raise my hand and slap her face in retaliation. I'm not proud of this, but it's the truth. I have worried about this response and have decided that it must be a basic human instinct, some primal self-defence reflex action from a time before humans evolved any sense of how to behave in polite society. Although . . . I have seen that nurse a few times in the supermarket since then and I still feel a tiny frisson of aggression towards her. Perhaps I am not fully evolved.

R is for results

Waiting for the results of your breast surgery and ANC (see page 10) is a kind of limbo. A dark and scary place: the borderland of hell. But remember, being at the gates of hell and actually being in hell are two very different things. Until you are told there is no hope, you must continue to hope. I had heard stories of women pestering the doctor for their results, unable to sit out the week-long wait to the review clinic. I wasn't so impatient. The way I saw it, for one week only I did not have cancer. For one week I was free to sleep and recover. My cancer was in a bucket in a lab somewhere. Next week they could tell me anything, but for that week I was cancer-free. I felt a bit high.

Then the morning of the results dawned and my reprieve was over. I was terrified. Hell awaited; and how cold it was. I could not stop shivering. By the time I reached the consul-tant's room I was shivering so much I was having trouble controlling the shaking. I'd brought a thank-you card for the doctor and ended up hurling it at her like a surly teenager. But I wasn't begrudging; I just couldn't get full control. I had to work really hard to sit still and hear what the doctor said: important stuff about grades and sizes and oestrogen and, of course, nodes. They recommend that you take someone with you to this meeting. I took a friend, but made her wait out-side the room. I am a big girl; I had to hear this news alone. The consultant smiled and said it was bad news because it was cancer, but it was good news because the tumours were small, ER positive and the disease hadn't spread. I was beside myself, and apart from flinging a card at her, I have no idea if I even thanked the woman.

Going to that meeting alone made me feel like cancer had not totally infantilised me. And it meant I had a moment alone with the news before sharing it with the world.

However, they are right. You do need support at this point. Which is why, before going in, I'd asked the breast care nurse if she would go over the details of the consultation with me and my friend later. She very kindly agreed. I also asked her to help me write down what the consultant had said. I definitely recommend this. It will give you a reliable record you can go back to; and if you are anything like me, you'll need it – I was already doubting the reality of this news before I'd reached my own front door.

As soon as I got my results I wanted to drive straight to my son's school and take him out of class and eat cake and cry. I did the cake eating and the crying, but I left the son in school. You will have to be really disciplined at this point. If, like me, you have led your child to believe there is nothing much wrong with you, you can't suddenly start celebrating your dramatic change in fortune. The child is bound to smell a rat and suspect your treachery, so that instead of reassuring them, you could end up worrying them unnecessarily.

When the reality of my results did finally sink in, I was hit by an overwhelming feeling of guilt. Others on the ward hadn't been so lucky; my cousin had been admitted to hospital because of a fever during her chemotherapy. I couldn't get any of these women out of my head. Why were they more sick than me? How could I face them? What fresh hell was this, when even good news was a torment?

A few weeks later I saw the breast care nurse again and

blubbed out how I was feeling. She didn't seem too surprised and that in itself was a comfort. She told me to concentrate on getting better and leave the others to her. She was right. Your guilt will help no one.

R is for radiotherapy

Radiotherapy is a weird mix of blinding technology and blinding simplicity. I was told some boffin in a lab is involved in working out exactly how much and where to pinpoint the radiation, and then your doctor comes along to measure and mark the relevant area on your body. I shivered as I lay on the bed, naked from the waist up, thinking, This is it: into your hands I commend my boob . . . And then he took out a ruler and a pen and proceeded to draw on me! It really was that lo-tech. I nearly burst out laughing, but I managed to control myself.

After the ruler-and-pen stuff though, the rest is all very Dr Who. All light beams and big machines and invisible killer rays. There is even a light beam that goes across the 'doorway' when you are being treated, so if someone should accidentally stumble into the room, they will be detected and the radiation will automatically shut down. Very sci-fi. The ten-year-old would've loved it.

Having radiotherapy is a bit like having an extended X-ray. Every day. For five weeks. You must remain completely still while you are being treated for fear that healthy tissue will get zapped. The radiotherapists tell you there is nothing to be frightened of, then promptly leave the room through a doorway that has a great big yellow and black danger sign above it. One time, I accidentally moved (the slightest movement) and the machine had to be stopped so that I could be repositioned. It felt like a lot of fuss and I burst into tears. But I wasn't crying in annoyance; I was crying at the reality of how dangerous radiotherapy actually is. That slight movement meant so much.

Radiotherapy *is* dangerous, but it is also amazing. I am constantly in awe of how scientists can harness forces like this and make them do what they want. I was seriously impressed that my radiotherapy burns had such precise corners, and took comfort knowing they could target areas so accurately without laying a custom-made stencil over me. So while radiotherapy is dangerous and does carry risks, you have to keep reminding yourself that many thousands of people are treated with it every year and they are OK. So why not you?

All of the radiotherapists I met were really nice and very professional. What's more, they did everything they could to accommodate me with convenient time slots for my treatment. You could not dislike them ... but I did wish they could have *talked me through* what was happening. You know, the way you tell a baby you are just changing its nappy even though you know it doesn't understand, or bellow at an elderly person, 'I'm just fixing your cushions,' when it's as plain as day that's what you're doing. Because the trouble with radiotherapy is that it isn't as plain as day. This enormous scary thing is happening and no one explains how it works. I did try to ask, but I suppose they just thought the answer was too complicated – all electrons and photons and ions and I wouldn't understand. Well that may be so, but couldn't they just try me?

Amazingly, for such a busy department, there were very few delays. These people are seriously efficient. Only rarely did I have to wait, and then my mind wandered: if I was very lucky, I might get turned into a superhero. Radiation gave Spiderman his superpowers, so why not me? (I do live with a ten-year-old boy, remember.) My powers would be unique: I would fly low over the world curing cancer at every turn. I would have a very nice leotard and a flat stomach. Then my buzzer would sound; time for treatment. Back to reality.

Note: radiotherapy makes you cry. This is odd because they don't cut you as in surgery, they don't inject you as in chemo and they don't give you pills as with hormonal therapy. The machine doesn't even touch you, and yet it is such an ordeal. Maybe it is precisely the fact that there is no obvious contact that makes it so unsettling. The rays are killing parts of you and yet you can't see or hear or feel them. Luckily, I had been warned about the crying effect by a friend, so when I blubbed once or twice it was a comfort to know that I wasn't the only one.

See also X is for X-ray.

S is for screening

I have an admission to make: I hate the word tits. Ugh, so vulgar. But sometimes there's nothing else for it, you have to call a tit a tit. Regular screening for breast cancer is offered to women between the ages of fifty and seventy.* Tough tits on the over-seventies. Really tough, since approximately a third of all breast cancers occur in this group. My aunt was in her seventies when she was discovered to have breast cancer; I was forty-five when I was diagnosed. So both of us were outside the screening brackets. Sadly, my aunt died, and I can't help thinking that things would be different for a lot of older women like her, if only they were screened. And I don't even want to think what could have been if I hadn't found that lump myself, but I am not complaining. All

---

*For some reason the upper age limit for screening in Northern Ireland was sixty-four until March 2009 when the health minister announced that this would be extended to include women up to the age of seventy. He reckons it will save lives. So do I.

screening programmes have to have a cut-off point. They have to target the group *most* at risk and apparently breast tissue is often too dense in the under-fifties for mammograms always to be effective. So screening is available, but it isn't perfect. If you are under fifty or over seventy, I suggest you take up hypochondria as a hobby. Mine finally paid off.

I thought everyone agreed that breast cancer screening was a good thing, but there has been some debate in the media recently about its usefulness. Only last week I listened to a radio programme where two men debated if we women were being mis-served by overscreening and overtreatment of breast cancers. The argument went that many pre-cancerous cells never become invasive and so could be left alone, but the screening process highlights these and selects women for potentially unnecessary cycles of surgery, drugs and radiation. I say *humbug* to that. I understand their argument, but I don't think the NHS spends money on unnecessary treatments (remember the storm over the cost of Herceptin?).

It doesn't take a genius to figure this out: screening can lead to early diagnosis and early treatment, and therefore a greater chance of being 'cured'. So keep checking and going for screening, I say. Because, to use my current favourite cliché, *better safe than sorry*.

S is for sick pay

Statutory sick pay runs out after twenty-eight weeks. If, after that time, you are still unable to return to work, you can apply for something called Employment and Support Allowance (ESA). This is a complex procedure: first of all your employer fills out a seven-page form informing the government of your status. Then, *you* fill out an eighteen-page form informing them of your status. (It is recommended that you do this over the phone as the form is complicated and offputting – it takes about half an hour.) Then the ESA people write to you asking for sick notes from your doctor confirming your status, and then for payslips confirming your pay. Then, when you've done all that, they send you a thirty-page form to fill out, yeah, you got it, confirming your status. How many different forms does it take to communicate, *I have breast cancer, I am on half pay, please help*!

My advice to you is get someone to help you with the forms (Macmillan and the CAB are helpful). Then be *very* patient and do not give up. The process can take weeks. But when that precious £60 a week finally arrived it was like a godsend. (See also Resources, page 213.)

S is for support groups

When my son was three and came home from nursery school with nits, I rejoiced. A child with nits is a child with friends; he wasn't standing in a corner on his own. You would be a rat to rejoice at anyone's cancer, but you can take comfort from the fact that you need never be alone again. Your family may be far away and you may feel that you don't want to burden friends any more, but you do not have to suffer alone. There are support groups out there focused on your cancer, and you can also make friends and find support at other activities run for patients such as yoga and relaxation, art or writing therapies.

I have only one problem with support groups: I hated the idea of being surrounded by people with cancer. If this sounds like you, I urge you to try and put your concerns aside, even for a short while. I did. I went along to a few support events and met other women in the same boat. Had I not ventured forth, I would never have met the woman whose cancer had returned, which meant that she had had to have two lots of surgery and radiotherapy. And yet there she was – larger than life. An inspiration. There is a lot to be said for seeing others who've come out the other side, and an uncomfortable comfort in knowing you are not alone.

S is for self-pity

Like setting your affairs in order (see page 14), I recommend you do self-pity early and quickly. It is impossible not to feel self-pity at a diagnosis of cancer, and you are right to do so because it isn't fair. It should be the wife beater, the murderer, the rapist, not you. You are right, so feel sorry for yourself and cry and let everyone know how sorry you are, then put it away before it threatens to drown you. You will need your strength, and for that reason feelings like anger and anxiety and self-pity have to be closely monitored. They can sap your strength at a time when you need it most.

S is for statistics

Oncologists love statistics. Thank God my GP warned me, otherwise I'd have been blinded by them. Following surgery, the oncology registrar told me statistical outcomes for my survival, then went on to tell me the statistics with chemotherapy factored in, then with hormonal therapy and, finally, with chemotherapy *and* hormonal therapy taken together. That's a lot of numbers, and maths not being my strong suit, I was really struggling with them.

There was a base figure which seemed to improve each

time another treatment was factored in. Great. I kept mentally totting up all the statistics I was presented with until I had reached the point where I was more likely to win the lottery than get cancer again. But of course, I wasn't a statistical anomaly; I'd done the sums wrong. And that brings me back to that adage from my old history teacher: knowledge without understanding is a dangerous thing.

They used a computer program called Adjuvant Online to estimate the risk of cancer mortality and the possible benefits and impact of the various treatments offered. The results were displayed in brightly coloured bands on the computer screen. I know this because a few days after my first oncology consultation I was still confused and upset, so I went, red-eyed and snotty-nosed, to my very nice breast care nurse who showed me the results and explained them in plain English. The doctor hadn't let me see the computer screen, which was very frustrating for me because I understand things better when I see them in writing (and no, I didn't ask – but then I didn't ask the nurse either). So I am grateful to the nurse who spelled it all out, and to my GP for warning me of the statistical snowstorm in advance.

I'm beginning to think that this 'statistics' consultation must be the one where the cancer patient finally cracks – freaking out crying and shouting at the doctor to *say it isn't so*, because the registrar I met looked almost as worried as I did. My figures were good, but maybe even good statistics are bad when it's cancer you're talking about, because instead of saying, 'Yay! Your prognosis is brill,' he adopted such a solemn tone that I thought he was about to pronounce me dead. He made a very sombre speech about there being statistics and would I be someone who would like to hear those. After his speech I naturally assumed the statistics were going to be bad (why else would he have used his undertaker's voice?), but I screwed my courage to the sticking place (as Lady Macbeth would say) and told him yes, I did want to know the statistics. I really only said yes because I hate people knowing things about me that I don't, but I am really glad I did. If I hadn't, I might not have realised that my prognosis was really very good. But it was a struggle to get at this information because of the doctor's worried look.

I later discovered that they have a policy of not offering chemotherapy to people for whom the benefit is less than 2 per cent. I came in at 1.9 per cent. I cried tears of relief when I found this out – no poisonous chemicals for me. But then I thought, 0.1 per cent? that's close! Shouldn't they give me chemo anyway, just to be on the safe side? But the computer said no.

So according to the computer, my prognosis was good, though you'd never have guessed it from the strained expression on the face of the registrar. I hope I'm not being too hard on him because he was very young and maybe he was almost as nervous as I was. Or maybe, like me, he didn't really trust the statistics. That's the trouble with computer-generated stats. Human frailty being what it is, you can't help wondering ... Is that program accurate? Which version are they using? Does the strapped-for-cash NHS keep abreast of advances in computer technology? I certainly hope the program is more reliable than the computerised diagnostic tool I use in my work to determine how much support students will need. It often throws up results that I know intuitively to be wrong. I then have to go to old-fashioned, non-computerised methods to prove the point.

My problem with statistics is that they are just that, statistics. Imagine you are the tallest girl in the class and proud of it. Then the teacher goes and works out the average height of the class and it comes in several inches short of your splendid altitude. You'd be pretty hacked off. The statistic accurately represents the class, but it does not accurately represent you.

So if the doctor gives you statistics that you don't like, don't despair. You are not a statistic. You are an individual. And while we're on the subject of statistics, here are some that might comfort you:

- In the 1970s around five in ten women with breast cancer survived the disease beyond five years; now it's more than eight in ten.
- Women diagnosed with breast cancer are now twice as

likely to survive their disease for at least ten years than those diagnosed forty years ago.
- Almost two in three women with breast cancer now survive their disease beyond twenty years.*

Good to know.

S is for sex

I've gone right off it.

S is for stereotype

There really is no escaping the clichés (see page 30) and stereotypes when you are sick. Everyone knows the stereotype of the arrogant-but-brilliant doctor. Don't pretend you don't. You can't tune into a hospital drama without being confronted by one. And it's been going on for decades: remember that bossy chap with the beard from the *Carry On* movies? And stereotypes of nurses also abound, from the caring

*Figures from http://www.cancerresearch.org.

Florence Nightingale types to the promiscuous, sex-starved, naughty girls in too-tight uniforms. Similarly, everyone knows the stereotype of the uppity patient who thinks they know better than their doctors.

I hate stereotypes and I hate being stereotyped. So when I hear people speak about their doctors in terms of the 'God complex', I cringe. And when I hear of know-it-all patients who arrogantly dismiss their doctor's advice, I feel a bit cross. I think we all need to learn a little humility and step outside the stereotypes.

But we also have to recognise that stereotypes exist because once upon a time there was more than a grain of truth in them. Sometimes there still is. Not all Irish men are the stereotypical drunks the media portrays, but some are. Not all female schoolteachers are frustrated spinsters with only a cat for company, but some are. Not all single mothers live off the dole in a council flat, but some do. Not all doctors fit their stereotype either, but some do.

So maybe the stereotypes and the clichés are unavoidable. And maybe we all have a need to simplify and package the world into known units, even if those units don't quite fit. Sometimes it's just easier. It's easier to believe that being deferred to makes doctors arrogant than to bother to look beyond the surface of what we see. But if we did, maybe we would see that some doctors appear aloof because it is the only way they can keep their distance and their sanity. Maybe they seem a bit cold sometimes because the alternative is to wade waist high through a valley of tears each day. Or maybe they really are just arrogant! But if they are, it has possibly more to do with their personality than their job.

I've met quite a number of doctors since starting my cancer treatment and few of them fit easily into any one stereotype. Some were kind and attentive and sensitive and informative. One was even funny too. Interestingly, many of these were in surgery (breast, bowel and gynae) – and surgeons are notoriously portrayed in the media as having a God complex. In fact, the bowel surgeon managed to be a complete gent, even while sticking a camera up my rear end.

So you see, sometimes the stereotypes are all wrong. And I am right to hate them. Some of the doctors I met were not stereotypical at all; they were atypically brilliant. I couldn't possibly speak for the ones I didn't meet.

T is for trust

Medicine is science not religion, but you still have to have faith. You have to believe that the doctor before you knows what is best. You have to have faith in the treatments that are offered. They have worked for others, they can work for you.

When you have cancer you need desperately to believe. But faith is one thing; blind faith is another.

The days when doctors were held in awe and unquestioned reverence are gone. If you prick them, they bleed. They are just like you and me. And you literally lay your life in their hands. If you are anything like me, you will want them to prove themselves worthy, show that they can be trusted. And that's a tall order, if you cannot actually see them . . .

When I asked why the radiotherapy consultant didn't come and see me, I was told he didn't need to. Maybe not, but I needed to see him. I needed to see him and hear him and know him. At least once. I needed to be told by this expert that he knew all about me – that he knew what the problem was and was going to fix me. But I didn't get to meet the man. Instead, I was told that treatment was standard, yet tailored to the individual. The dose of radiation would be accurately determined by measurements taken from the surface area of my breast, my lung volume, etc. I had nothing to worry about; the physicist would work it out.

Well, here's the thing: I am not an equation. I am a human being who was terrified. I needed that doctor to reassure me. And I'm not talking about a pat on the arm and a smile. My consultant surgeon isn't a bit touchy-feely, but she is visible at all times. I've seen her at all but one appointment. I see how she cares about her work. She has always been there, taking control, taking *responsibility*, and so I had no problem handing myself over to her for the chop. I trust her.

My radiotherapy consultant, no doubt, had many patients to see who were much worse off than me (though presumably, so did my surgeon and my oncologist). He may have been attending important meetings or writing a crucial paper on radiotherapy to the breast area, or doing any number of vital things that I could never even begin to understand. These people are busy. I get that. But, somehow, they need to make time to meet with us. Call me precious if you like, but I believe that we have to learn to trust these people, and I believe that they have to earn that trust. It is not a given.

This whole idea of trust is central to the cancer experience. You must trust, you must *believe*. But it can all start to sound a bit silly after a while. I keep waiting for someone to point the finger at me and whisper fervently, 'Verily, I say unto thee, believe and thou shalt be cured.' It's all bound up with the idea of Positive Mental Attitude (PMA – see page 138). You have to go grinning like a goon into your treatment if you want to have any chance of coming out alive at the other end. You must never let your PMA flag for a second. You must not dissent. You are letting the side down if you do. I have felt this acutely from the start. To question, to have doubts or concerns, is frowned upon. You are being negative, and we all know where that leads.

I think maybe we have such a tenuous hold on our health

and our futures at this time that it makes us all a bit desperate. Of course, being positive is important, but honestly, I sometimes felt like I was trapped with a bunch of evangelists *praisin' the lawd* who looked at me askance if, like Doubting Thomas, I dared to say *show me*.

And the awful thing is that even when you do believe and you do trust your doctors, you can no longer trust your own body. How could it have played this rotten trick on you? One day you were perfectly healthy, trusting without thinking that you'd be here and be healthy for years to come, the next, you have a killer inside you. And you just can't help thinking, How long was it dormant? And then, once you've been treated, How long will it be before the beast reawakens? So that every time you bleed or don't bleed, every time you ache, every time your heart pounds, every time you feel some new pain inside you, you falter. Your body is not to be trusted. It is a trickster, mocking you, making you fearful and wary, always on the lookout. Hunted.

I don't know how you start to trust your body again. I'm not there yet. I'll just have to put my faith in clichés and trust that time will heal.

T is for touch

Never before have my breasts been so much on display and touched by so many different hands. Yet no one is really touching me; they are touching a wound, a cancer site, a reconstruction. They are not touching *me*. About three months into my treatment I felt this acutely. I felt like my body was an object to be poked and examined. A sick curiosity. I am not complaining; this had to happen. But I sat down and cried because I desperately wanted someone to touch me as a person, not as a cancer patient. I needed basic physical contact like I have never needed it before in my life. So, thank you to the friends who just sat and held my hand or put an arm around me and said absolutely nothing when I cried.

Go out and hug someone today.

PS I've just found out that, interestingly, some cancer charities offer 'touch' therapies. So I'm not the only one.

T is for tea

A few years ago I read in the newspapers that tea can help prevent cancer. Brilliant. Next to wine it is my favourite drink.

Apparently, tea is full of the antioxidants that help fight free radicals – these are not political extremists, but the molecules that damage cells and can lead to cancer. What a great excuse to sit down and put your feet up. It has to be proper tea mind you, not a mean old teabag dunked in a cup. It should be made in a pot and left to draw properly. Just the way I like it.

There was also a news story around the same time as the tea one claiming that the theobromine in dark chocolate is actually good for you too. Bingo! A cup of tea and a chocolate biscuit: just what the doctor ordered.

I decided to check all this out and found a cache of websites that told me tea could prevent cancer – and just as many that told me *hot* tea could increase my risk of throat cancer. Honestly, how are you supposed to find your way through this maze? There is so much information about what you can and can't eat, which foods contain antioxidants, which *type* of tea you should be drinking. You could become very confused and just a teensy bit obsessed. And some people do – completely changing their diet and lifestyle, cutting out dairy, alcohol and meat, etc. I am not going to do this. I refuse to be condemned to a life of Quorn and soya milk.

Don't expect your habits to change overnight just because you have been given a diagnosis of cancer, but do try slowly to introduce changes to your regime. I started by making sure I had the five a day. Then I took a temporary pledge not to drink any alcohol for as long as it took me to write this A to Z and just to see what being teetotal would be like. (It is boring; roll on Z.) To paraphrase the late great Clement Freud, giving up drinking doesn't make you live longer; it just seems longer.

T is for tissue expander

This is an inflatable implant which sits underneath the chest muscle. It has a small metal port through which saline is injected over a period of weeks. This isn't as hair-raising as you'd think. In fact, I think it looks worse to the bystander because one nurse said to me, 'I'd have run. I don't know how you did that.' But I didn't *do* anything. I was prodded and poked a bit and then the needle went in. You have to remember the breast tissue has been removed and the needle doesn't have to penetrate too deep before it hits the metal. It is uncomfortable and inexplicably tiring, but it is not painful. Each time the 'bag' is inflated, your skin stretches slightly, giving the impression of a breast. Sometimes the doctors had difficulty injecting the saline into mine. At other times I left the clinic with a plumped-up half boob and would be delighted until a few days later I noticed that the thing had deflated slightly. To be honest, the tissue expander is more disc-like than breast-like, but it does the job. And eventually, it is removed and a permanent implant inserted, which I am told will give a more realistic shape.

Tissue expanders are ideal if you have small breasts because you can get a near-symmetrical look fairly quickly. It can also make the mastectomy psychologically easier to deal with because from day one and thereafter you will have a small mound where your breast was. So the feeling of loss is alleviated.

It is uncomfortable to begin with because the chest muscle doesn't like the alien intruder and sometimes goes into small spasms when you exert yourself. I would be a liar if I said that having a piece of metal and a bag of liquid in my chest wasn't weird, and I admit to a whole new set of worries: Christ! What if it bursts – will I drown? Would the piece of metal mean I'd fry during radiotherapy, like tinfoil in a microwave? I was too embarrassed to ask the first of these questions, but the answer to the second is no. (Don't ask why. Nobody said.)

All this work on the boob meant that I was sore for quite a long time, so the ten-year-old needed an explanation as to why he couldn't just jump up and hug me spontaneously. I knew he'd be fascinated by the technology, so I told him a bit about the implant. 'Can it burst?' was his first question. (I should have taken him along as my cancer buddy and he could have asked all the questions I felt too foolish to broach.) I also told him that I had a piece of metal inside me which the surgeon located with a magnet. His eyes widened, then he ran out of the room, and I thought, Oh God, too much information. I went too far that time. He returned a minute later with the strongest magnet he could find and held it close to my chest until he could feel the force, 'Cool,' he said. 'You'll beep going through airports.'

Yeah, cool.

I've heard that people dislike tissue expanders because they involve such a long, drawn-out process. I didn't mind. I think it gives you time to adjust. And I have loads of time: the final part of my reconstruction has been set back for a while, so I will have spent over a year with my almost-boob. If I were an artist like Tracey Emin I might take casts of the different-shaped boobs I'll be sporting over this year and exhibit them at Tate Modern. I could pile every bra I've ever worn in the middle of the floor – a lamentation or celebration of a past (I would let the viewer decide which because I wouldn't want to be too prescriptive). I would call it 'Every boob I've ever slept with'. Hmm, now that's got me thinking ... Wonder what Damien Formaldehyde Hirst would do? But I'm not Damien Hirst or Tracey Emin. I'm me, and I will sit it out.

Work in progress, as the artists say.

T is for telephone calls

Your telephone bill will rocket. I soon found I was phoning people during the most expensive part of the day because my son was safely tucked away at school and wouldn't overhear anxious snippets of conversations about cancer. Even if you have been open and told your children, grown-up conversations can still frighten them. My phone bill almost trebled during this time and I sat around chewing my nails about this for months. All I had to do was contact the phone company and change my package to suit, but it seemed like such a big job. It is very easy to let your finances get on top of you at a time like this. You might be lucky enough to have a partner or husband to look after this side of things, but if not, grasp the nettle. The longer you leave these things, the worse they will get.

At the beginning, when I was first diagnosed, I felt under siege; my phone never stopped ringing. At times I found myself wanting to pull it from its socket, just to get some peace. Three months later, my phone barely rang and I found myself checking the socket to see if it was plugged in correctly. I asked around and know that I am not alone in this. So don't feel too bad if you think people have forgotten you. It's just the way of the world.

U is for unsung heroes

What about a big cheer for all those hospital folk who don't ever get the limelight? I'm thinking of the diagnostic radiologists, the anaesthetists and the poor benighted lab workers. You may never actually meet any of these people, and yet their contribution to your survival is crucial.

While lying in hospital recovering from my mastectomy, I did sometimes wonder about my disembodied boob and those all-important lymph nodes. When people asked me how I was, I remember saying I was great because my cancer was in a bucket in a lab somewhere, not anywhere near me. However, I did often worry about how exact and focused these lab workers need to be, how deadly serious their job is: mix up those petri dishes and we're all done for.

And then there's the anaesthetist. If he or she doesn't get their job right, your surgeon doesn't stand a chance. Just having an anaesthetic is potentially highly dangerous. On the few occasions when I've had to undergo surgery and medical staff have asked me if I am aware of the risks of an operation I've always thought, Yeah, the anaesthetic could kill me. But who ever thinks to send a thank-you card to the anaesthetist?

And while I'm at it, what about the clerks and secretaries who label and file and sort us all out? Just think: one slip from them and who knows where you'd end up. The surgeons get the glory and the glamour, but they are at the top of a pyramid made up of many disparate, and often no less important staff. So spare a thought for these sometimes unseen and often unsung heroes.

U is for unreality

An hour or so after I had told my mother about my cancer and imminent mastectomy, I managed once again to convince myself that I had made the whole thing up. I drove home berating myself: I really had to stop lying like this. What kind of attention-seeking insanity had taken hold of me? I genuinely felt as though I had lied and that the cancer was just one great big mistake. I told my GP this and she said, 'That must be the unreality people talk about with cancer.' It is as if this awful thing is not really happening to you. I have heard of some people feeling as if they are *watching* it happening to them, almost like an out-of-body experience; others move like automatons, not really engaging with the process. I suppose it is the mind coping and not coping.

Even when your breast has been removed and you have the stitches to prove it, when radiotherapy has left its mark across your chest and chemotherapy has made all your hair fall out, you may still not quite believe that you are sick. When I suggested to one woman who had just finished her chemotherapy and was about to start her radiotherapy that she might be entitled to financial help in the form of Disability Living Allowance she said, 'But don't you have to be sick for that?' My reaction exactly. Bizarrely, I thought she should be entitled to it and she thought I should, but neither of us thought we were entitled ourselves.

Now, a full six months on from diagnosis, when trying to sort out sick pay or insurance or my job, I still baulk when asked the reason for my absence from work. Then I say cancer and I still don't believe it. I see it written on a sick note or a letter from the hospital and cannot attach the word to myself. Cancer is something that happens to other people. This cannot be real.

U is for uncertainty

This much is certain: after cancer, uncertainty is a fact of life. Get used to it. No doctor will tell you your cancer has gone for good; no matter how good your prognosis, no doctor will pronounce you cured. The threat will always exist and you have to live with it. Your friends and family may forget. They will see you 'getting on with life' or 'getting back to normal' and assume you too have forgotten. But of course you won't have. There is no normal now, because you had cancer. You could have died, but you didn't. And you can't even properly rejoice in case you tempt fate and the bastard comes back to bite you.

One doctor told me that I had statistically nearly as much chance of dying from my cancer as I had from some other cause like a road traffic accident. I told the ten-year-old and we laughed: I would never cross the road again. If only it were that simple. There is nothing you can do to guarantee your cancer will not return. And you simply have to get used to this because you still have to live in the world.

I have to pretend I am 'back to normal' because that is what everyone wants to see. This is hard because cancer has sucked out all my confidence. I am cowed and wary and aged now. I cannot believe that once I stood before people and spoke with confidence, or had the audacity to hold an opinion, or chat up a stranger in a pub. And I cannot believe I will ever do these things again. One friend tells me that we get confidence from doing things and that when I am back at work 'doing things' and socialising again my confidence will return. Maybe she is right. The one thing I have not lost my confidence in is being a parent. Perhaps because I never stopped doing it.

This loss of confidence is complicated. It can't just be put down to no longer having two boobs; I bet people who have non-breast-related cancers also undergo this crisis. I think it is down to the fact that something fundamental changes when you are told you have cancer: all your certainty is stripped away. And I think it is as basic as this: once I dreamed of the future, of all the things I would do and see my son do, and then one day the future was snatched away from me. My prognosis is good. They have given me the future back, but I saw into a world that did not include me and the picture will not go away. So I start making plans, but they seem hollow, risky, built on sand. And that fear will be with me always. This is the fact of cancer. But instead of sitting around moping, use it to your advantage. The genie has granted you one power: the ability to love the moment you are in. Sometimes, I forget I had cancer. Until I remember. Use the memory to enjoy the here and the now.

U is for universe (centre of)

Six months after my operation I went into a public swimming pool at peak time sporting only one and a bit boobs and no prosthesis. I know that for relatively flat-chested women like me this is easier, but it still isn't easy.

I chose my costume carefully. Bypassing the skimpy, spaghetti-strap bikinis with a sigh, I chose a boring one-piece swimsuit that came up almost to the collarbone and had enough padding to hide my one nipple joke. It was one of those serious swimsuits that flattens even the perkiest of breasts. Streamlining you. I was sure to knock a few seconds off my lap time.

I stood at the tunnel entrance of the pool (you know, where you have to step through a shower) and wondered how I would make it to the safety of the water. I felt like I was in one of those awful anxiety dreams where you find yourself at work with no clothes on and can't figure out how to get home unnoticed. People brushed past me, impatient and eager, and I made my move. My instinct was to cower and scuttle to the edge of the pool, but I thought I might look like a pervert or a weirdo, so I stood up straight and walked like a normal person. And the strangest thing happened: no one turned to gawp. No one even batted an eyelid. No one noticed me. It seems I am not the centre of the universe.

Tip: if you are anxious about your skin reacting with the chlorine, smear the affected area with ointment like Vaseline or Diprobase. It will act as a barrier and prevent the area from drying out. It worked for me. You might feel like you're being smeared with goose fat in readiness to swim the Channel, but it'll be worth it. I later sewed my softie prosthesis into my swimsuit and finally found a good home for it.

And please note: I waited months before I went swimming. You have to be careful with radiotherapy skin, so ask your doctor first.

V is for valid

Let no one make you feel that your cancer, or your reaction to it, is not valid. Some people may find the force of your emotion overwhelming, and so end up trivialising the whole experience in an attempt to 'lighten things up'. They will make your mastectomy and reconstruction sound like a boob job; they will make radiotherapy seem like a trip to a tanning salon. And I have lost count of the amount of times I heard the words, 'You are only having radiotherapy.' They obviously hadn't heard correctly; I said *radio*therapy, not *aroma*therapy.

Probably, these people were only expressing relief that I didn't have to go through chemo, but these other treatments are a big deal too: surgery and hormone treatment and radiotherapy can leave you shaken. But that's not the point. Even if radiotherapy is the one type of treatment you receive, *only* is the wrong word. Last week I sat opposite a woman who told me about her cancer diagnosis and said that she'd *only* had a hysterectomy. *Only*, I squawked at her. *Only*? I felt like crying. She was a youngish woman and after repeatedly reporting symptoms to her doctor, she was finally taken seriously and investigated. Too late to save her womb. She had no children and I didn't ask if this had been through choice. I hope so.

I too have found myself saying, 'I *only* had ...' and somehow the implication is that my experience is less valid than others': I am not entitled to the full range of support or sympathy on offer. There are loads worse off. So there are, but if you are ever made to feel like this, just think of that woman and her hysterectomy and know that your experience is real. Your feelings are valid.

V is for visiting time

You'd think I'd absolutely hate being in hospital, but there was one thing I really loved: visiting time. Once a day I would comb my hair, put my make-up on and sit in the visitors' room to wait. Visitors are not allowed to sit on the beds, so if I was going to get a hug from the ten-year-old, I needed to be in position. He soon got the hang of it. I could be hugged on one side, but not the other. Each day he would come in, smile and put his arms around me and we would sit in quiet adoration of each other. A silent mutual-appreciation society. It was heaven. Maybe in reality this only lasted a few minutes, but it seemed to me like a blissful eternity.

Otherwise, I know from experience that hospital visiting times can be fraught. For both the patient and the visitor. Expectations are high, and everyone feels the need to have something interesting to say – but of course, you won't (unless you think discussing your compression stockings is interesting). And to make things worse, visitors worry about tiring you and you worry about tiring them. It's tricky.

I only had a few visitors because I only told a few people that I was in hospital. I see now that this put them under pressure to do all the visiting, so maybe it wasn't such a good idea. One nurse noted my lack of visitors and said I was denying myself support, but in a way, I can now see I was also denying those friends I had told support too. Another argument in favour of full disclosure (see D is for disclosure and H is for honesty).

W is for waiting

Waiting is part and parcel of cancer. Waiting for tests, waiting for results, waiting your turn ... I've heard some people say this wearied them, but on balance, I felt content to wait. The staff were busy – many clinics have standing room only – and you just have to prepare yourself for the long haul. After a while, you should become inured to it. But it is hard going when you are exhausted from treatment or your concentration is so poor that you can't pass the time reading.

Once I had to wait a *very* long time and when finally I was seen, the staff said to me, 'Why didn't you complain?' I said, 'Well, no one likes a whinger, do they?' But it wasn't just that – where cancer is concerned you can't help wondering if the person before you has a more worrying, more scary cancer than yours. Maybe some poor soul is desolate and staring death in the eye, and the staff can't prise themselves away. You can hardly complain, can you? You just have to accept it, because in the words of Henry Van Dyke:

> Time is
> Too Slow for those who Wait,
> Too Swift for those who Fear.
> From *Music and Other Poems*

You can't have it both ways, so be patient.

See also R is for Results.

W is for wildfire

Once you've uttered the words 'I have cancer', the news will spread like wildfire and you can't fight it, so don't even try. I wore myself out trying to swear people to a vow of silence and then checking constantly that they still hadn't told. Unless your friends happen to be Trappist monks, you will have to face the reality that they will most likely tell someone. Married/partnered friends are the trickiest. As a single woman, I confess that I am more than mildly irritated by the way 'attached' friends feel they have a right to share with their partners what I have shared with them. It drives me mad. I am not shy; if I wanted to tell my friends' husbands the intimate details of my life, I would. If I ask friends not to tell their husbands about my cancer, I'm not being disingenuous. I mean it. Desperately. Mostly, because I'm terrified their children will overhear (and they might, in turn, tell my son their Chinese whispers version of events), and partly because I can only deal with the enormity of this in tiny little slices. It's not that I don't understand. I was in a relationship long enough to remember the relief of offloading and getting comfort, so I am really, seriously impressed with the many friends who respected my need for privacy when they really wanted to have a good cry with their husbands.

One of my friends tells me she thinks it ridiculous that I would ask someone in a relationship to keep a secret like this from their partner. She also reckons that given similar circumstances, I would probably spill the beans to my partner if I had one. Then, as if to prove my contrariness, one woman (also having breast cancer treatment) told me how upset she became when her husband told the neighbour about her cancer. She was livid – hadn't she specifically asked him not to? I listened patiently and nodded sagely. I understood perfectly. But I also understood the husband. Of course he was going to tell the neighbours. What did she expect?

It occurs to me that the problem has largely to do with deciding who gets told and when. I suppose it is really about control. Until I had told my son about the cancer, I was desperately trying to control the flow of information so that it wouldn't reach him before I was ready. And what a job that was – like trying to put out wildfire with a water pistol. So maybe my friend is right. Maybe you shouldn't dare to hope that news like this could ever stay secret. I don't know. But I do know that insisting on secrecy, as I did, only adds to everyone's stress. So take it from me: don't do it.

W is for waterproof mascara

This will feel as if you are applying liquid bitumen to your lashes, but if you cry as much as I did and don't want to look like a trollop who doesn't wash her face after a night on the town, then it is essential. Waterproof mascara looks just as effective as regular mascara – and it really works; trouble is, it is the devil to get off. After extensive research I recommend Johnson's baby oil on a cotton-wool pad. Works a treat and is far cheaper than any fancy eye make-up removers that claim to remove even waterproof mascara. Go on, cry your eyes out.

W is for work

You will hear stories of how some people kept on working throughout their cancer treatment. Honestly, apart from the obvious problem of fatigue, these people need to go easier on themselves. This is not the time to be defined by your work. I appreciate that it may help take your mind off your worries, but it's a fine line between distraction and denial. You are sick; you are entitled to time off – take it. Even if you have a really cool job, the chances are you'll be too tired to do it anyway.

My advice is to spend time being sick now and save time later. I know of a woman who worked all through her breast cancer treatment: surgery, chemo and radiotherapy. A real Trojan. Then treatment stopped and everything just went on as normal and the poor woman crumbled. She became really anxious and depressed and felt she couldn't cope any longer. Worse still, she found herself revisiting and recounting her treatment to anyone who would listen. But by this stage most people were looking at her sideways thinking, Well you're OK now, aren't you? What's the big deal? If only she had been easier on herself all along, others would have seen that she needed help and time to be sick.

When you have been diagnosed with cancer you are protected by the Disability Discrimination Act, which means that you have a right to expect your employers to accommodate any reasonable needs you have and that includes being allowed time to be sick and to get better. Smaller employers may not know this, and larger, unscrupulous employers may pretend they don't, so be warned: you could have to fight for your rights. The Act also offers you some protection if faced with dismissal or redundancy. This last issue preoccupies me. They can't sack you, but they can clear your desk and dump all your stuff in a bin bag (thanks guys) ...

In any event, when you are sick, this is the time to be good to yourself. Take it easy, have a lie-in. Don't be a superhero – just get well.

NB If you are worried that you are being unfairly treated because of your cancer, contact the Equality Commission or any disability rights group. They can help.

W is for weight

I thought cancer was some kind of wasting disease, so how come I've gone up a dress size in six months? And unless shoe shops are deliberately mislabelling their goods, even my feet have put on weight. Seriously, I've gone from shoe size 39 to 40. Perversely, my remaining boob has stubbornly remained the same size, while annoyingly, fatty tissue on the side I was operated on seems to have migrated to under my arm and I now have bra overhang on that side. If this keeps up, I will become one of those flat-chested fat women who can find nothing to wear. I am not impressed. I have been a vain size 10 for about three decades and in recent years had started to get smug about it. Is this hubris then, Tamoxifen or just the cake with custard I took to eating to see me through radiotherapy?

X is for X-ray

The ten-year-old told me that X-rays were discovered accidentally in 1895 by the German scientist Röntgen. Apparently, he was working on another experiment when he noticed strange rays in the room and not knowing what they were, he called them 'X'. He then took a picture of his wife's hand using the rays and saw her bones – and the rest is history. (I wonder if the bit about the wife's hand is true. Probably.)

A week or so after telling me about the origins of X-rays my son informed me of another husband-and-wife double act: the Curies. He explained how they discovered radium and that it could be used to treat cancer. Ordinarily, I wouldn't worry about my son relaying these little nuggets to me. He does it all the time, like a house cat proudly laying dead mice at my back door, but when he added, 'Marie Curie died of radiation poisoning in the end,' I began to worry. Was he concerned that I would come to harm? Should I hide those *Horrible Science* books he's so addicted to? I quizzed him about this, and found, to my relief, that he was more interested in the fact that the Curies worked on deadly substances in their garden shed and that the radiation burned a hole in Mr Curie's trousers than any possible relevance this may have to boring old me. Well, I wouldn't be carrying any radium around in my pockets, so that was all right.

Unlike my son, there is a huge science-shaped hole in my education. Physics clashed with history and I was doomed. I thought quark was a cheese spread until my son told me that they – quarks – are subatomic particles. He was only about eight at the time, so when he told me their names (up, down, charmed, strange, bottom and top) I thought he was making it up, until I checked the dictionary. Clearly I am science illiterate, so I had no idea what these doctors were doing to me. I desperately wanted to understand, but the received wisdom seems to be that it's all either too complicated or too scary for patients to digest. All they would tell me was that X-rays and other strong rays would kill the cancer cells, but would let the healthy cells live. Honestly. This kind of non-explanation just made me more confused and more frustrated. It sounded like a primary school approach to religion to me: *we shall smite*

down the bad cells and let the good cells go forth and multiply.
I needed more.

By the time I started my radiotherapy treatment I had discovered that it can give you cancer, damage your heart, lungs, bones and skin, but when I said that I was worried, people just looked at me like I was a silly old fusspot! Eventually, about three weeks into my treatment, a registrar took note of my frustration and sat down and drew me a rudimentary diagram illustrating cell cycles for cancer and for healthy cells, explaining that they divide and repair at different speeds, and some other complicated stuff that I'm afraid to repeat in case I get it wrong. Anyway, he managed to convince me that radiotherapy wasn't just space-age witch-doctoring, and a little bit of trust came creeping back.

Trust or no trust, I was having this treatment and I just had to get on with it. I was told that I might get some mild sunburn effects, like reddening and soreness; I might become breathless and I'd feel tired from all the cell repair going on inside me. A friend told me that the hair in my armpit would fall out, so in the interests of symmetry I began shaving the other armpit again. What is it with cancer and hair? Does hair behave like cancer cells and therefore get killed off in the same way? (More great unanswered questions. See how I am constantly tormented by my own ignorance?)

Anyway, the fact is that doctors are not fortune tellers. They do not have a crystal ball, so they cannot predict how you will react to treatment. However, they do know what is *possible* and they can prepare you for this. And I believe that if you know what is coming, you are better able to deal with it. A great deal of my anxiety was caused by not really knowing what to expect. I know doctors don't want to alarm patients, but sometimes forewarned is forearmed.

My skin started to react to the treatment during my second week of radiotherapy and I was confused. The information I received suggested that a reaction might occur towards the end of weeks three or four and that it is more likely to happen to the very fair-skinned (I'm not fair). By the fourth and fifth weeks my skin was burning hot all the time and had turned a purple-black in the armpit. And it got worse, but I won't burden you with the details except to say that I assumed a new nickname: Chernobyl Chest. The cool gel pads the nurses gave me to ease the pain simply curled up and fell off with the heat. I was on fire. The ten-year-old amused himself checking the heat from my skin at various distances. We joked about making toast at it. But I wasn't really laughing. Sunburn-like effects? Yeah right – maybe if you went out in the Sahara at midday and forgot your factor 150.

Confused, I read and reread the radiotherapy leaflets. But none of the information I'd been given described the burns I had. Did that mean that mine were outside the norm? I panicked. Was skin cancer the next stop on my 'journey' (see page 116)? If I'd done this to myself through a bout of extreme sunbathing, I'd be berated for my foolishness. And I'd stop. But the radiotherapy didn't stop. Instead, the radiotherapists now carefully laid clingfilm over my chest to (I assume) stop my ragged skin tearing off on to the equipment; the nurses gently washed and dressed the wound every day; and I still didn't get to see that consultant. So I could only assume that burns of this nature were normal. But if that was the case, why didn't it say so in the information leaflets?

Eventually, when radiotherapy was almost at an end, one of the radiotherapists explained that the Superflab (a cushion of gel set on top of my skin during treatment) had probably made me burn more severely. Why couldn't they have told me that at the start when I asked? '*Super – flab*? Really? What does that do?'

I spoke to other women who were undergoing radiotherapy too, but none of them had a skin reaction like I did, so hopefully you won't either. I was just unlucky, it seems. And what luck: my bedroom was like a clinic, full of creams and saline tubes and dressings. It was too painful to shower properly or sleep easily, but my distress was caused as much by worry and ignorance as by the physical discomfort.

But I'm better now. My bedroom is cleared of dressings and creams. My skin has healed and hopefully the radiotherapy has done its job. The whole area is scarred from the burns and they tell me this will never go away, so I won't be modelling my armpit any time soon. But so what? That won't kill me.

See also R is for radiotherapy.

Y is for youth

I used to like my doctors like my wine: aged. I wanted them to be at least the same age as me, preferably a bit older, but as I get older I realise that this is just not viable.

Don't be too dismayed if the registrars look like they are twelve. They aren't really getting younger; we are getting older. When the surgical registrar came round to see me before my operation I took fright. Surely this young bucko wouldn't perform the operation! I know these young doctors have to learn and they have to learn by doing, but all I could think was, Please don't learn on me. Please just watch this time round and write an essay on the experience: a thousand words on the advantages of a full mastectomy over a lumpectomy. Yet youth has never been a deterrent to brilliance and sometimes it is a boon. That new young doctor may be full of bright ideas, up to date with the latest developments; they may be energetic and enthusiastic.

Consider your own workplace. Think about those who are

about to retire – some are conscientiously grafting away to the bitter end, taking pride in their work the same way they have always done, while others are coasting and counting the days to retirement. Now think of the younger workers in the organisation. Some are lazy clock watchers, cutting corners; others are hardworking, conscientious and dedicated. Doctors are no different. They have frailties and faults just like the rest of us. Take each doctor as an individual and give the bright young sparks a chance.

And there are advantages to being seen by a young doctor: because of your advanced years (remember, I was all of forty-five when this started) they may hold you in as much reverence as they do their own granny. This has the effect of making them really *very* polite and respectful. I experienced this once and I have to admit it was kind of cute, even if it did make me feel ancient. And there are other benefits too. Sometimes it is the less experienced doctors who talk more openly to you or say something an older doctor would be far too guarded to utter. One young doctor said to me, 'If I was going to have cancer, I'd want yours.' I felt quite flattered and a bit smug, as though I'd been clever enough to get a *good* cancer. An older, more experienced doctor might not have said that to me, and I would've missed out on that prickly comfort of knowing that things could be a whole hell of a lot worse.

Y is for y me?

This is a pointless question. It is you. Give it up.

Z is for ZZzzs

One month into motherhood I remember saying that what I wanted more than anything was to go to bed one night and wake up the next morning. Simple as that. Four weeks of night feeds and nappies had left me wrung out and the idea of an unbroken night's sleep had become nirvana. I became obsessed with the amount of zeds I was getting and even used to keep a little tally each night so that I could compare it with my fellow new mothers. After the babies, sleep was our favourite topic of conversation. I thought I would never have a night's sleep ever again. But I did.

With cancer, the broken nights came back, but bleaker this time round. I stopped sleeping through the night on the day I was diagnosed. Sleeping tablets were recommended; insomnia, it seems, is part of the deal. I woke in the small hours to despair and silent tears. I dozed and woke again before dawn, only to begin crying all over again. My pillow was soaked. Then treatment started and I moved seamlessly from insomnia to somnambulance.

Suddenly, I felt like I was sleepwalking through my own life. I could not keep my eyes open. If I sat down for a moment to listen to the radio or try to read the paper, I would nod off, but perversely my nights were still broken. This narcolepsy was frustrating for me and boring for the ten-year-old. Any joint activity we engaged in – from chess to channel hopping – culminated in me snoozing. I even fell asleep in the viewing gallery at the pool while watching his swimming lesson (he was not impressed).

When I wasn't trying to go to sleep I was trying to stay awake. I was in a muddle for months before I realised that cancer makes you tired even when you can sleep. Everything about the treatment impacts on your energy levels: surgery and anaesthetics make you tired, hormonal therapy makes you tired, chemotherapy makes you tired, radiotherapy makes you tired, the anxiety of having all or any of these makes you tired. And frustratingly, no amount of sleeping seems to make you less tired. So try not to languish around too much as this will add to the feeling of lethargy and will only make matters worse: you will be like a sloth crawling through your own life.

They recommend going for short walks as this offers the dual benefit of giving an instant spurt of energy and a delayed sense of exhaustion, hopefully, just in time for bed. (Trouble is, most of the time I was too bloody knackered to go for a walk.) They also say you should allow yourself a little extra sleep, but not too much. I usually found that a timed granny-nap after lunch would just about keep me going until bedtime. I would set the alarm on my mobile phone and lie on the couch. You are allowed to be tired, so let it happen. Who else gets to go for guilt-free zzzzs in the middle of the day?

All this sleeping and not sleeping means you can get very little done. I would have a sleepless night and be drained all day. I would start on a task and before I knew it, bed would be calling me. I started to write this A to Z during my radiotherapy treatment but, as I told a friend at the time, I couldn't get past A because I kept falling asleep. After the radiotherapy ended, I set myself a target and pushed myself to stay awake a while longer every day until eventually the nap was mostly abandoned. But even then I could not conceive of a day spent at work or any other activity without the option of a nap. Impossible.

Fortunately, I had to get the ten-year-old off to school, so I had to get up every morning like a normal person. This routine helped; otherwise, I might have been having breakfast during *Blue Peter*. Sometimes I found I was so drained I couldn't bear to cook dinner and would have gone to bed hungry were it not for Oliver Twist looking up at me wanting a proper meal.

If only being tired like this guarantees you a night's sleep, but insomnia is a cruel master. The things that scared you at the beginning still scare you. Has the cancer really gone? Will it come back? What are these drugs doing to my body – will a hysterectomy really be necessary? Did I tell my son too much or not enough? And that's just the cancer. Then there are all the other things that keep you awake at night, like being on half pay and wondering who to rob this time round, Peter or Paul; fussing over which secondary school to choose; worrying about how long my bed-bound father could last without eating properly. And then there was always next door's crying baby . . .

And of course, you will be tired of just *thinking* about cancer. But one day you will realise that you have not thought of cancer for a whole hour, a morning, an entire day. You do not have to live cancer all the time. Your cancer diagnosis won't go away, because the day you were diagnosed your life changed for ever. But remember, while cancer may shape you, it doesn't have to define you. You do not have to be the victim or the survivor. You can just be. And one night you might even lie down to sleep and miraculously wake to find it is the next morning.

Epilogue

R is for recovery

The day after I was diagnosed with cancer I was in Boots the Chemist when the idea for this A to Z came to me. I stood there with a basket in my hand, blinking back tears and thinking, Now, what does a breast cancer patient need? All I could come up with was waterproof mascara. I put one in my basket and thought, Someone should write an alternative guide to breast cancer – Step one: buy waterproof mascara; you're going to need it.

A few short months later, I found I was writing the guide myself. In between hospital appointments, I sat in bed with my laptop, furiously, desperately, trying to make sense of this alien world I had entered. I felt a bit crazed – the nutty professor naming and labelling things: A is for ... I suppose it was my way of trying to impose some order. Nothing made sense any more and writing this book was like having a conversation with myself, trying to understand what was happening; a daily pep talk to keep me sane, to keep me going, to make me feel like I still had some control.

A lot of time has passed since I wrote this book. I am nearing that longed-for five-year milestone, and already I see changes in the world of cancer. I read in the papers that Tamoxifen may now be given to women who are at risk of cancer, but who have not yet developed the disease. And I understand that lymph-node removal can now be avoided with a procedure called sentinel lymph-node biopsy, whereby they only check the sentinel nodes and, as a result, many women are spared the risk of lymphoedema. (I checked sentinel in the dictionary – it said, 'A soldier or guard whose job is to stand and keep watch.' Cool, huh?)

And a lot has happened to me, most significantly the deaths of both my parents. But I am still here. I have outlived them, and that is as it should be. Still, I feel saddened reading the small references to them.

What strikes me most though on reading this book now is how frightened and ignorant I was. But it is the anger that chills me the most. In the movies cancer victims always seems so sweet and accepting. They embrace the monster and make their peace with it. Remember Susan Sarandon in *Stepmom*? Not only did she accept her cancer, but she accepted Julia Roberts as a replacement 'mom' for her children. Insult to injury. You'd never catch me doing a thing like that. Cancer didn't make me come over all Zen, it didn't turn me into a Care Bear; it turned me into Mrs Angry. Now, when I look back on that time, it is with relief that I am not that person any more, but still I make no apologies for it. You'd be a pretty odd fish not to feel angry about having cancer. But you have to let it go some time, otherwise you'll just get stuck in a groove, and then where would your Positive Mental Attitude be?

When I wrote this book I thought I would never confidently face the world again, but you know the old cliché, 'Time heals all wounds'? Well, it's true. Sort of. And a lot of time has passed since then. Time often spent in tears and turmoil. Yet here I am, *healed*. I've got my new boob, my wounds from surgery and radiotherapy have faded to small scars, my 'bad' arm only hurts sometimes and while the deadening fatigue proves difficult to shake off, my sleep has improved. But none of this was easy and none of it was quick.

One day while I was having physiotherapy on my arm, the nice, no-bullshit physiotherapist said to me, 'Recovery from cancer treatment can take years, you know.' *Years*! I nearly choked. Wasn't Kylie back strutting her stuff long before that? Years of this. I could have cried. But I didn't want the physiotherapist to decide that telling patients this kind of thing was a mistake. Yes, I was horrified, but I still needed to know. So I said nothing and filed that piece of information away for a rainy day. And I am glad I did, because I was able to go back to it whenever I needed reassurance – whenever I felt I wasn't 'back on track' like so many you hear about: the ones who run marathons while having chemo; who work full time, manage their families and climb Mount Kilimanjaro for charity in their spare time. That wasn't me. I crawled through the days, struggling with fatigue and my emotions and the horror of going back to work. Thank God that physiotherapist let me know that recovery can take so very long. So don't be alarmed. Getting over cancer takes time. I only started to see light at the end of the tunnel after I'd passed the halfway post to that all important five-year marker.

Time does heal, slowly, by degrees. But it does not travel backward. Nothing can erase the assault that is cancer. There will always be a part of me that is afraid, but that part is shrinking.

'So, tell the truth,' my son says to me. 'When are you going into hospital again?' It seems he too is fearful.

I cannot tell him never. How do I know what lies in store? How do any of us? Like me, he just has to accept that this is how it is. I may get sick, I may not. I might live until I'm ninety or I might step out smiling one day, right into the path of that double-decker bus. Who knows? He tells me that Marie Curie's husband Pierre died in an accident: after years of working with radioactive substances, he was killed when he fell under a cart in the street.

Life and death really are so very random. That's hard to

accept when you are a seasoned worrier like me. Worriers don't like random. As a teenager, already frustrated by my flair for worrying, I bought a cartoon postcard of a stick-man worrier. Stick man becomes so concerned for his own safety that he locks himself indoors and, eventually, just stays in bed, safe and sound. Until a spring comes loose from his mattress and stabs him in the heart. 'Death by Mattress' the cartoon was called. After you've had cancer taking a risk can seem harder than ever, but you have to try. So when you falter, let this be your mantra: *beware of death by mattress.*

While I was having my cancer treatment life seemed to me like a trick – a gift given in error that might be snatched back at any moment. I put all my plans on hold and put all my energy into holding on. All this time later, here I am. Still holding on. Sometimes I feel like I owe my life to the nurses and doctors who helped me, and sometimes I think I owe it to me. I found the lump. I reported it when I really wanted to pretend it wasn't there. I faced up to what might happen. I did what I had to. I am alive. I am here. And already just being alive is no longer enough. I have plans.

Resources

www.cancerfocusni.org
Cancer Focus Northern Ireland provides information and help across a whole range of cancers, as well as specific help to people experiencing breast cancer, including an excellent post-surgery bra-and-swimwear fitting service. They offer a range of complementary therapies and have an excellent counselling service. They also run a family support facility to help children deal with the cancer diagnosis of a parent/loved one. I especially found their free information and support line invaluable (0800 7833339); it offers help to patients, friends and family alike.

www.cancerresearchuk.org
I found this website most useful for information on the lymphatic system. It is clear and uncluttered and the diagrams are simple and easy to understand. Go to *About breast cancer – The breasts and lymphatic system.*

It is also brilliant for explaining the reconstruction process. Go to *About breast cancer – Breast reconstruction using implants.*

www.breastcancercare.org.uk
This is especially useful for help with coping emotionally, and deals with the problem of body image and worrying about self-esteem after surgery. It also has a great downloadable factsheet on reducing the risk of lymphoedema:
http://www.breastcancercare.org.uk/upload/pdf/Web_Reducing _risk_lymphoedema.pdf

www.breakthrough.org.uk
This website has an excellent video and illustrations to help you understand how to self-check your breasts. Go to *About breast cancer/touch-look-check.*

www.macmillan.org.uk
Macmillan has a full and comprehensive website about all cancers, but I found it useful for checking through possible treatments, especially for information on Tamoxifen and hormone therapies. There is a good section on risk factors and how diet and lifestyle may be related to cancer. They also have some excellent images of breast and even nipple reconstruction.

The site also includes a good, clear overview of Disability Living Allowance and Employment & Support Allowance, with useful telephone numbers. Go to *Cancer information – Living with and after cancer – Financial issues – Benefits and financial help.*

Otherwise, for non-health-specific issues the following organisations are helpful:

www.equalityhumanrights.com and www.equalityni.org
For when things get bad at work: advice and information for people experiencing discrimination following a cancer diagnosis. They will give you clear and concise information on the Disability Discrimination Act 1995, which now covers cancer.

www.disabilityaction.org
This site offers specific advice and support for getting back to work in Northern Ireland. I found them invaluable.

**www.healthwatch.co.uk and
www.patientclientcouncil.hscni.net**
These organisations (telephone 0300 0683000 and 0800 9170222 respectively) can offer assistance and advocacy for cancer patients who are experiencing problems or have complaints about their care. They offer information in a range of languages.

Finally, for anyone interested, the science books that my son – and, in turn, I – read were *National Geographic Kids* and the *Horrible Science* series. Why didn't they have books like that when I was small?

Index